The Rehab Pocket Survival Guide

Scott Woska, MD

Other titles from International Medical Publishing
Clinician's Handbook of Preventive Services, 2nd edition
Guide to Clinical Preventive Services, 2nd edition
The sixth Report of the Joint National Committee on Prevention, Detection, Evaluation, and Treatment of High Blood Pressure

The Rehab Pocket Survival Guide is provided as an educational resource for trainers, physical therapists, and physicians. It is not a substitute for supervised training.

First Printing.

The Rehab Pocket Survival Guide
Scott Woska, M.D.
International Medical Publishing, Inc.

ISBN 1-58808-111-7
Price: $9.95

Order on the web from: www.medicalpublishing.com

Published by International Medical Publishing, Inc.
P.O. Box 479, McLean, VA 22101-0479
Phone (703) 356-2037 Fax (703) 734-8987
www.medicalpublishing.com

Printed in the United States of America

The Rehab Pocket Survival Guide

Scott Woska, M.D.

Chief Resident
Columbia University
College of Physicians and Surgeons
Columbia Presbyterian Medical Center
of the New York Presbyterian Hospital
Dept of Rehabilitation Medicine

This book is intended primarily as a reference for the busy Rehabilitation Resident in taking care of patients on the inpatient rehab unit as well as outpatient musculoskeletal and specialty clinics.

It may also be very useful for the resident in Neurology, Orthopaedics, Rheumatology, Neurosurgery, Geriatrics and Internal Medicine as well as for medical students and therapists.

The content is kept brief with the goal of highlighting the most important concepts and teaching points of the major rehabilitation topics in a portable and easy to use format. While it is used for quick reference, the reader is pointed toward the major textbooks and journals for more complete information.

Special thanks to Michelle Stern, M.D. for her review and suggestions.

Special thanks to my wife, Sharon, for her support and encouragement throughout the years.

Contents

III. Specific Disorders 35

IV. Diagnosis & Treatment of Pain 73

Introduction

PM&R or Physical medicine and rehabilitation became a specialty in 1947 by the American Board of Medical Specialties. The Physiatrist focuses on the whole person in a functional environment utilizing a team approach.

Interdisciplinary team

Resident	Attending	Rehab nurse
Social worker	Physical Therapist	Occupational Therapist
Speech Therapist	Psychologist	Vocational counselor
Prosthetist/orthetist	Nutritionist	Equipment vendor
Speech Pathologist	Recreational Therapist	

Impairment: Any loss or abnormality of psychological, physiological or anatomical structure or function.

↓ visual tracking	visual field loss	↓ visual acuity
↓ scanning	ideational apraxia	motor apraxia
body neglect	spatial neglect	topographical confusion
spatial dysfunction	agnosia	body scheme disorder
↓ attention	memory loss	impaired judgement
confusion	↓ alertness	distractibility
labile	postural dyscontrol	↓ limb control
proprioceptive loss	↓ endurance	balance loss
pain	weakness	sensory loss
↓ coordination	↓ ROM	spasticity

Disability: Any restriction or lack resulting from an impairment of the ability to perform an activity in the manner or within the range considered normal for a human being. – Inability to ambulate, perform ADLs

Handicap: A disadvantage for a given individual, resulting from an impairment or disability, that limits or prevents the fulfillment of a role that is normal for that individual.
Societal level – Wheelchair inaccessible

Physiatric History & Physical

CC HPI PMH PSH All Meds

Physiatric History Focus

Prior functional hx
Present functional level
Vocational hx: education
Avocational: hobbies, religion, support groups
SH: Living arrangement, environmental barriers, stairs (indoor & outdoor), w/c accessibility, doorway size, insurance, finances
FH: DM, CAD, CA, rheumatic disease, gout, CVA, kidney stones, HNP, neuromuscular disorders

ROS: DOE, exercise tolerance, claudication, swallowing, reflux, n/v, constipation, b/b continence, dysuria, frequency, hesitancy, voiding history, sexual function, pain, stiffness, cramps, deformity, memory, comprehension, speech, sensation, weakness, fall history, depression, skin problems

Physiatric Physical Exam Focus

Skin: integrity, discoloration, ulcers, groin folds, infection, scars, toe nails, callous, subcutaneous nodules
Rectal tone
Bladder palpation
Peripheral pulses, edema, calf tenderness
Spine curve, alignment, tenderness
Limb deformity, atrophy, length discrepancy, tender points
Joint stability, ROM, contractures

Neurological Exam: MMSE, speech, CN, strength, sensory, DTR, coordination, tone, bulk, RAM, gait
Waddell Criteria for non-organic LBP: Tenderness (superficial or non-anatomical), Stimulation (axial loading or rotation), Distraction (SLR), Regional (weakness, sensory), Overreaction (most important)

I
Physical Exam

Normal Joint Range of Motion

Cerv sp.	flex	60°
	ext	75°
	lat flex	45°
	rotation	80°
Shoulder	flexion	180°
	extension	60°
	abduction	180°
	int rot	70°
	ext rot	90°
Elbow	flexion	150°
Wrist	flex	80°
	ext	60°
	pron	80°
	sup	80°
	radial	20°
	ulnar	30°
<u>Thumb</u>		
CMC	abd	70°
MCP	flex	50°
IP	flex	80°
<u>Digits 2–5</u>		
MCP	flex	90°
	ext	20°
PIP	flex	100°
	ext	30°
DIP	flex	70°

Lumb sp.	flex	60°
	ext	25°
	lat flex	25°
	rotation	20°
Hip	flex	120°
	ext	30°
	abd	40°
	add	30°
	int rot	45°
	ext rot	45°
Knee	flex	140°
Ankle	dorsi	20°
	plantar	50°
Subtalar	inv.	30°
	ever	20°
<u>Toes</u>		
1st MTP	flex	30°
	ext	50°
2nd MTP	flex	30°
	ext	40°
3rd MTP	flex	20°
	ext	30°
4th MTP	flex	10°
	ext	20°
5th MTP	flex	10°
	ext	10°

Cervical Myotomes

Proximal nerves	C5	C6	C7	C8	T1
Rhomboids (DS)					
Supra/Infra spinatus (SS)					
Deltoid (Ax)					
Biceps brachii (MC)					
Radial Nerve					
Triceps					
Anconeus					
Brachioradialis					
Ext Carpi Radialis					
Ext Digitorum Communis					
Ext Carpi Ulnaris					
Ext Pollicis Brevis					
Ext Indicis Proprius					
Median Nerve					
Pronator Teres					
Flex Carpi Radialis					
Flex Pollicis Longus					
Pronator Quadratus					
Abductor Pollicis Brevis					
Ulnar Nerve					
Flex Carpi Ulnaris					
Flex Digitorum Profundus(med.)					
Abductor Digiti Minimi					
Adductor Pollicis					
1st Dorsal Interossei					

Adapted from Brown WF, Bolton CF: Clinical electromyography, ed 2. Boston, 1993, Butterworth-Heinemann, with permission.

Lumbosacral Myotomes

Proximal Nerves	L2	L3	L4	L5	S1	S2
Iliacus	■	■				
Adductor Longus (Obt)		■	■			
Vastus Lateralis/Medialis (Fem)		■	■			
Rectus Femoris (Fem)		■	■			
Tensor Fascia Lata (Sup Glut)				■	▒	
Gluteus Medius (Sup Glut)				■	▒	
Gluteus Maximus (Inf Glut)				▒	■	
Sciatic Nerve						
Semitendinosis/membranosis (Tib)				■		
Biceps Femoris - Short head (Per)					■	▒
Biceps Femoris – Long head (Tib)					■	▒
Peroneal Nerve						
Tibialis Anterior			■	■		
Extensor Hallucis			▒	■		
Peroneus Longus				■		
Extensor Digitorum Brevis				■	■	
Tibial Nerve						
Tibialis Posterior				■	▒	
Flexor Digitorum Longus				■	▒	
Gastroc Lateral				▒	■	
Gastroc Medial					■	▒
Soleus					■	■
Abductor Hallucis					■	■
Abductor Digiti Quinti Pedis					■	■

Adapted from Brown WF, Bolton CF: Clinical electromyography, ed 2. Boston, 1993, Butterworth-Heinemann.

Dermatomes

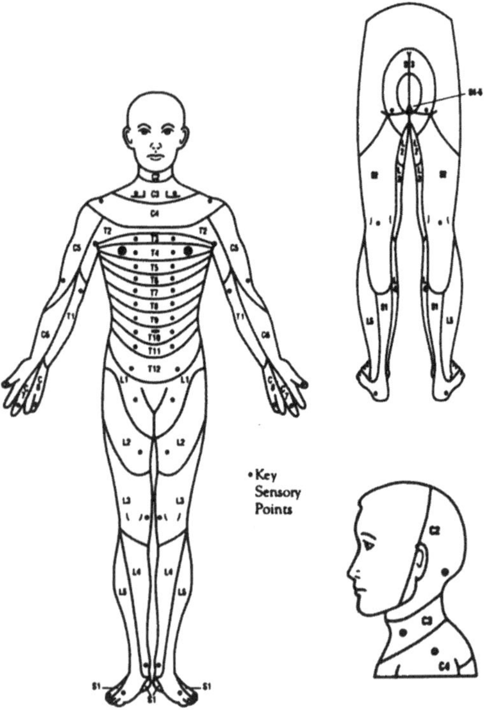

Reprinted with permission of American Spinal Injury, Association, Chicago, 1992 (from International Standards for Neurological and Functional Classification of Spinal Cord Injury).

Median Nerve

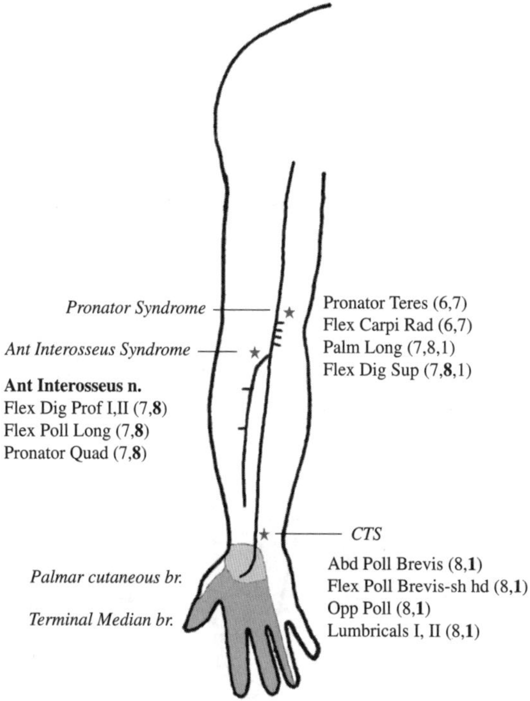

Ulnar Nerve

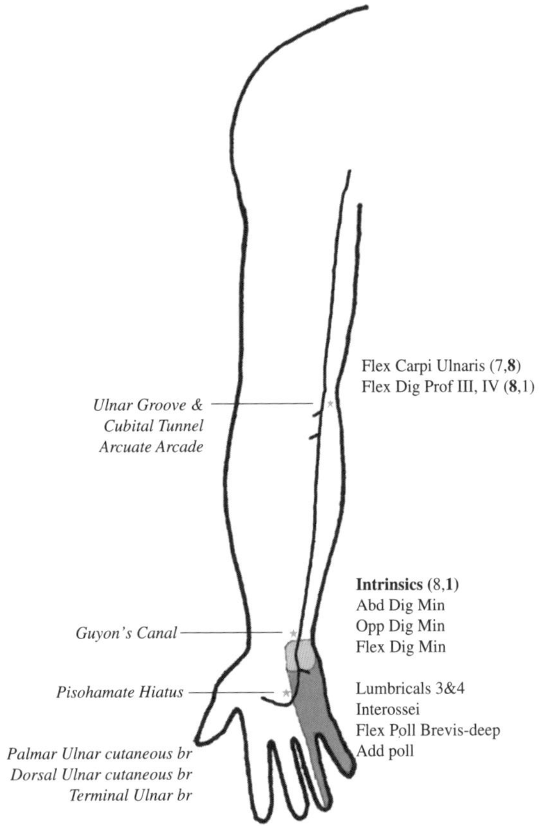
Flex Carpi Ulnaris (7,**8**)
Flex Dig Prof III, IV (**8**,1)
Ulnar Groove &
Cubital Tunnel
Arcuate Arcade
Intrinsics (8,**1**)
Abd Dig Min
Opp Dig Min
Flex Dig Min
Guyon's Canal
Lumbricals 3&4
Interossei
Flex Poll Brevis-deep
Add poll
Pisohamate Hiatus
Palmar Ulnar cutaneous br
Dorsal Ulnar cutaneous br
Terminal Ulnar br

Radial Nerve

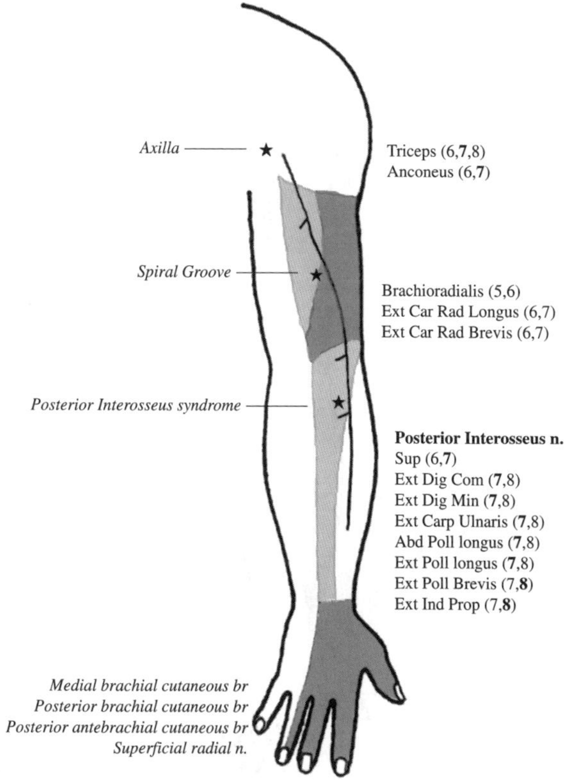

Axillary and Musculocutaneous Nerves

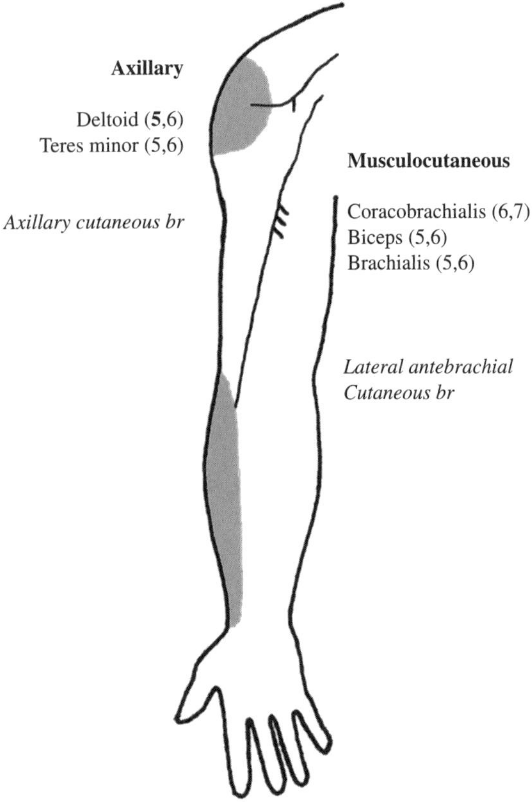

Brachial Plexus

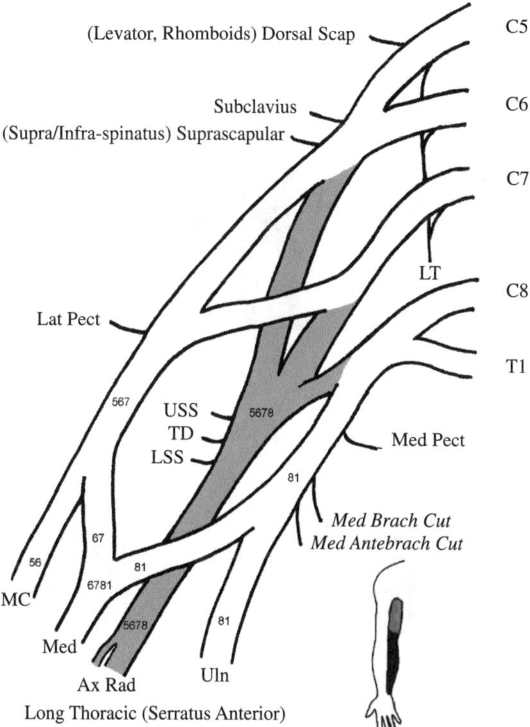

Long Thoracic (Serratus Anterior)
Upper & Lower Subscapular (Teres Major)
Thoracodorsal (Latissimus Dorsi)
Med & Lat Pect (Pectoralis Maj/Min)

Femoral and Obturator Nerve

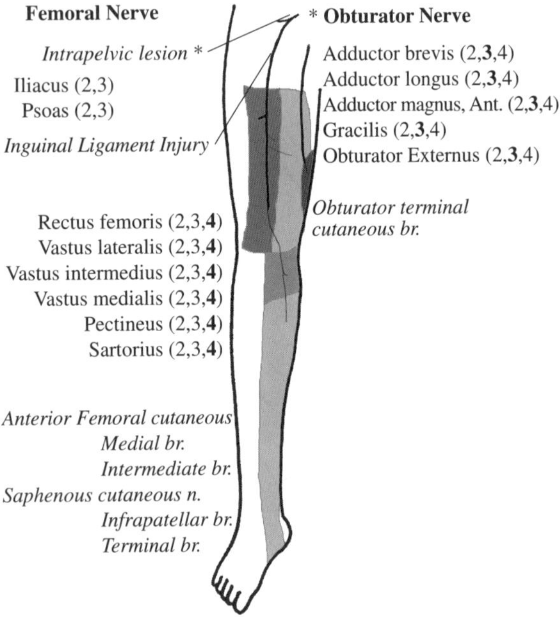

Sciatic, Tibial &Gluteal Nerves

Superior Gluteal Nerve
Gluteus Medius (4,**5**,1)
Gluteus Minimus (4,**5**,1)
TFL (4,**5**,1)

Inferior Gluteal Nerve
Gluteus Maximus (5,**1**,2)

Sciatic Nerve
Biceps, long hd (5,**1**,2)
Biceps, short hd (5,**1**,2)
Semitendinosis (**5**,1)
Semimembranosis (**5**,1)
Adductor Magnus, post.

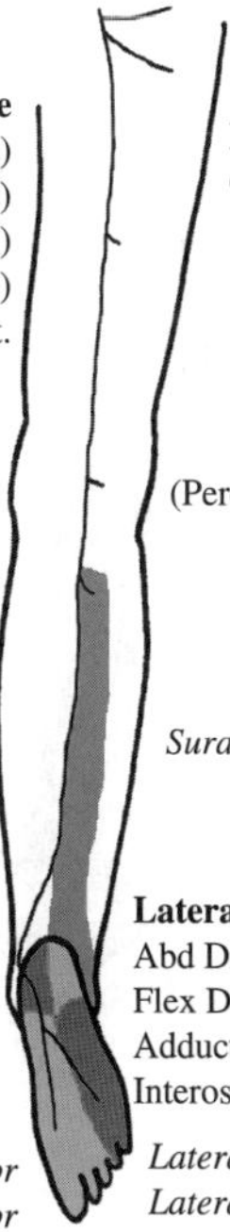

(Peroneal)

Tibal Nerve
Gastroc, med (**1**,2)
Gastroc, lat (5,**1**)
Soleus (1,2)
Tibialis Posterior (**5**,1)
Flex Dig Longus (**5**,1)
Flex Hallucis Long (5,**1**,**2**)
Popliteus (5,1)

Sural cutaneous nerve

Tarsal Tunnel *

Medial Plantar Nerve
Abd Hallucis (1,2)
Flex Dig Brevis (1,2)
Flex Hallucis Brevis (1,2)

Lateral Plantar Nerve
Abd Digiti Minimi (1,2)
Flex Digiti Minimi (1,2)
Adductor Hallucis (1,2)
Interossei (1,2)

Medial Calcaneal br
Medial Plantar br

Lateral Calcaneal br
Lateral Plantar br

Peroneal Nerve

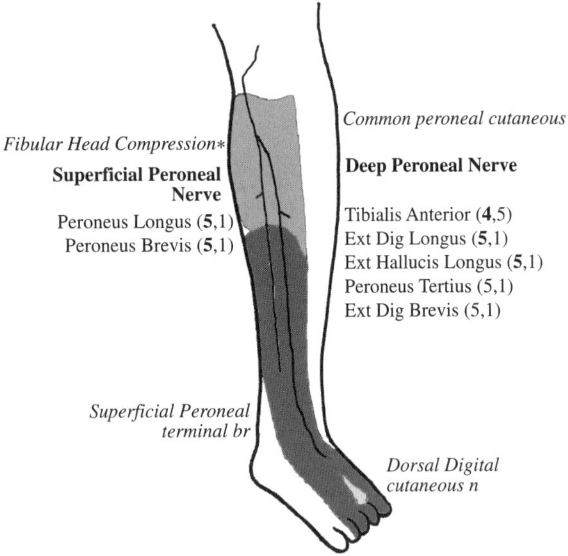

Lumbosacral Plexus

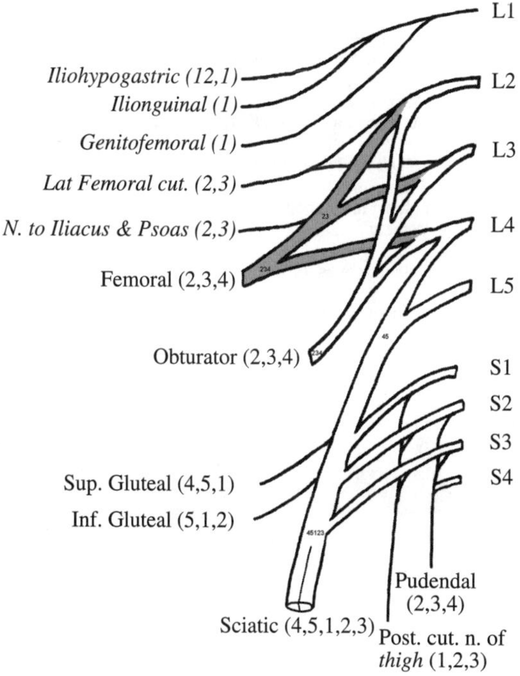

Manual Muscle Strength Testing

of Kendall, McCreary, and Provance

In Antigravity position holds test position against:

5	Strong pressure
4+	Moderate to strong pressure
4	Moderate pressure
4-	Slight to moderate pressure
3+	Slight pressure
3	No pressure
3-	No pressure with gradual release from position

In horizontal plane moves through complete range

2+	against resistance
2	Without resistance

In horizontal plane moves through partial range

2-	Without resistance

No movement with

1	Feeble contraction, prominent tendon
0	No visible contraction

Rancho Los Amigos

Levels of Cognitive Functioning

1 No response	Unresponsive
2 Generalized	nonspecific, non-purposeful
3 Localized	Specific, inconsistent
4 Confused, agitated	Incoherent
5 Confused, inappropriate	Alert, simple commands
6 Confused, appropriate	goal directed behavior
7 Automatic, appropriate	robot-like, supervision needed
8 Purposeful, appropriate	independent, carry over learning

Glasgow Coma Scale

Eye Opening	Spontaneous	E 4
	Response to speech	E 3
	Response to pain	E 2
	None	E 1
Best Motor Response	Obeys verbal commands	M 6
	Localizes pain stimulus	M 5
	Flexion withdrawal	M 4
	Abnormal flexion	M 3
	Extensor response	M 2
	None	M 1
Best verbal response	Oriented, conversive	V 5
	Disoriented, confused	V 4
	Inappropriate words	V 3
	Incomprehensible	V 2
	None	V 1

<8 severe   9–12 moderate   13–15 mild

Modified Ashworth Scale of Spasticity

0	Normal
1	Slight ↑ tone, catch and release Minimal resistance at end ROM
1+	Slight ↑ tone, catch Minimal resistance through remaining ROM
2	More marked ↑ tone through most of ROM
3	Considerable ↑ tone, passive movement difficult
4	Rigid

Synergy Patterns

	Flexion Synergy Components	**Extension Synergy Components**
Upper	Scapular retraction Shoulder abduction, external rotation **Elbow flexion** Forearm supination Wrist/digit flexion	Scapular protraction Shoulder Adduction, internal rotation Elbow extension **Forearm pronation** Wrist/digit flexion
Lower	**Hip flexion,** abduction, External rotation Knee flexion Ankle Dorsiflexion, inversion Toe dorsiflexion	Hip extension, adduction, Internal rotation **Knee Extension** **Ankle plantarflexion,** inversion Toe plantarflexion

Gait Analysis

The 6 determinants of gait: minimize displacement of the center of gravity,

Pelvic rotation	around vertical axis (4°)
Pelvic tilt	4° downward tilt during swing
Pelvic lateral displacement	
Knee flexion	at heel strike and heel off
Ankle dorsiflexion	during late stance
Knee-ankle-foot unit	coordinated movement through stance

Trendelenberg gait	glut med weakness, hip drops
Antalgic gait (asymmetric)	limit time in stance, hip hike & lean
"Waddling" gait	bil glut med weakness
Foot slap	weak DF (foot drop)
Genu recurvatum	Hyper extended knee 2° ↑ PF
Steppage gait	Excessive PF of good side
Circumduction	Excessive abduction in semi-circle
Hip hiking	Lift hip during swing

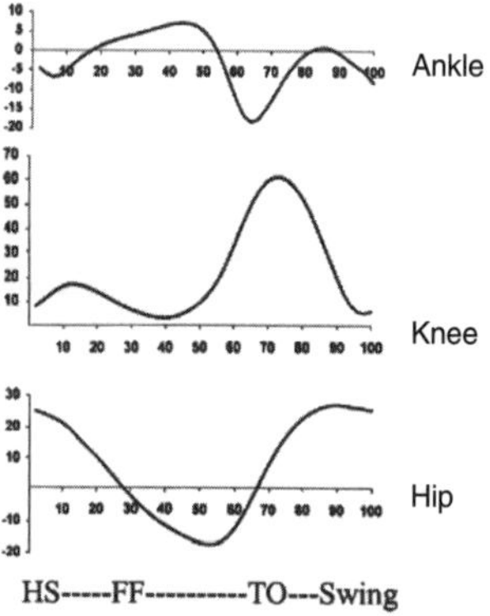

Center of Gravity = 5 cm anterior to S2

Average Gait velocity 80 m/min or 3 mph

Average cadence 70–130 steps/min

HS = Heel strike
FF = Foot flat
TO = Toe off

Functional Independence Measure – FIM scale

	Dep = Dependant
1	Max A = Maximum assistance
2	Mod A = Moderate assistance
3	Min A = Minimum assistance
4	CG = Contact Guard
5	CS = Close supervision
6	DS = Distant supervision
7	I = Independent

Self Care
- Eating
- Grooming
- Bathing
- Dressing UE
- Dressing LE
- Toileting

Sphincter Control
- Bladder
- Bowel

Transfers
- Bed, chair, w/c
- Toilet
- Tub, shower

Locomotion
- Walk, w/c
- Stairs

Communication
- Comprehension
- Expression

Social Cognition
- Social interaction
- Problem solving
- Memory

From Uniform Data System for Medical Rehabilitation (Adult FIM) version 4.0. Buffalo, NY, State University of New York, 1993 with permission.

Pulmonary Function Tests

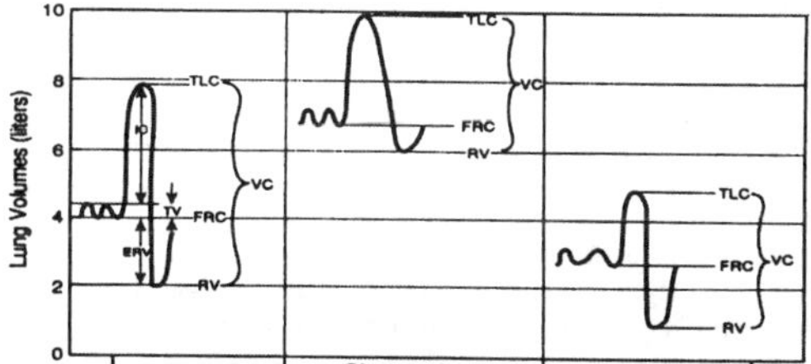

	Normal	Obstruction-hyperinflated	Restriction
VC (liters)	6.0	4.0	4.0
TLC (liters)	8.0	10.0	5.0
FRC (liters)	4.0	7.0	3.0
RV (liters)	2.0	6.0	1.0

(From Kelly WN: Textbook of internal medicine, ed 3, Philadelphia, 1997, Lippincott-Raven, p.2111; with permission)

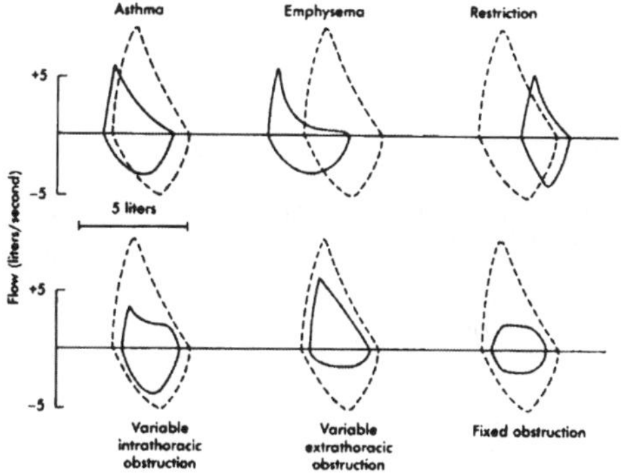

(From Ruppel GE: Manual of pulmonary function test, ed 6, St. Louis, 1994, Mosby, p.56; with permission)

Exercise Physiology

Aerobic capacity = the work capacity of an individual = VO_2 max
CO = HR X SV
mVO_2 = Myocardial O_2 consumption
VO_2 = Total body O_2 consumption
VO_2 Max = maximum O_2 consumption
RER or RQ (respiratory quotient) = VCO_2/VO_2 (efficiency)
AT = anaerobic threshold, when RQ=1
AT normally reached ~ 45–60% predicted VO2max
O_2 pulse = VO_2/HR
Predicted VO_2 max (sedentary middle age man) (ht-age) x 21
RPP = HR X SBP (indicates aerobic conditioning)

VE = volume of exhaled air (~3–4L during exercise)
MVV = max voluntary ventilation (forced breathing)
Resp reserve = MVV-VE

Intensity of exercise : (Max HR ~ 220-age)
Target HR 85% of max in normal patients
Target HR 60% of max in diseased patients
Cardiac benefits at 20–30 min 3–5x/week
Effects: ↑ aerobic capacity, CO ↑ at max exercise.

Low Level exercise (<50% max, aerobic)
- VE ↑ in proportion to VO_2
- Tidal volume ↑ more than resp rate
- Dead space/tidal volume ↓ from 0.3 to 0.1

Moderate level of exercise (>50% max, anaerobic)
- VE ↑ out of proportion to VO_2
- Resp rate ↑ rapidly, tidal volume plateaus.

Maximum exercise (Near VO_2 max)
- <85% total lung capacity
- Dead space/tidal volume <0.1, RR ~ 50
- PaO_2 & $PaCO_2$ maintained near normal
- Arterial lactate ↑ >0.4 mmol/ml

MET Table

Activity	METs
Lying quietly	1.0
Sitting at ease	1.2-1.6
Sitting writing	1.9-2.2
Standing at ease	1.4-2.0
Walking 1 mph	2.3
Standing and washing	2.5
Standing and dressing	2.3-3.3
Light housework	1.7-3.0
Heavy housework	3.0-6.0
Office work	1.3-2.5
Walking 2 mph	3.1
Light industrial work	2.0-5.0
Walking 3 mph	4.3

MET = energy demand of a given activity estimate

1 MET = 3.5 ml O_2/Kg/min

Multiply number of METs by 3.5 to get VO_2 for that activity for an average person, however actual values vary

Borg's Rating of Perceived Exertion

6	
7	Very very light
8	
9	Very light
10	
11	Fairly light
12	
13	Somewhat hard
14	
15	Hard
16	
17	Very hard
18	
19	Very very hard
20	

Category-Ratio Scale (CR-10)

0	Nothing
0.5	Extremely weak
1	Very weak
2	Weak
3	Moderate
4	Somewhat strong
5	Strong
6	
7	Very Strong
8	
9	
10	Extremely strong

Mini Mental Status Exam

Score	Orientation
5	What is the (year)(season)(date)(day)(month)
5	Where are we: (state)(country)(city)(hospital)(floor)
	Registration
3	Name 3 objects (i.e. apple, table, penny) Give 1 point for each correct answer
	Attention and calculation
5	Serial 7's backwards. 1 point for each correct answer Alternately, spell "WORLD" backwards 1 point for each correct letter
	Recall
3	Ask for 3 objects repeated above 1 point for each correct answer (Note: Recall cannot be tested if all 3 objects were not remembered during registration.)
	Language
2	Name a "pencil" and "watch"
1	Repeat "No ifs, ands, or buts"
3	Follow a 3-step command "Take a paper in you right hand, fold it in half and put it on the floor."
1	Read and obey the following: "Close your eyes"
1	Write a sentence.
1	Copy the design:

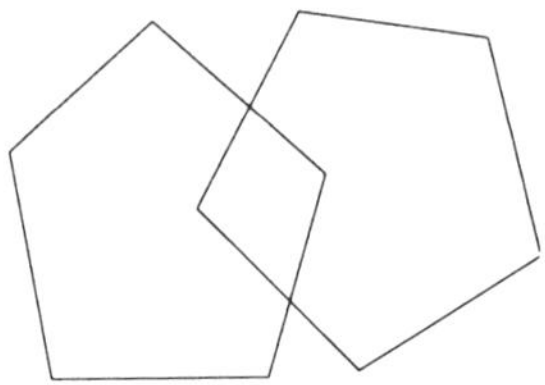

Total

Mild impairment >21 Moderate impairment 10–20 Severe impairment <9

Aphasia Algorithm

Fluent

Good Comprehension	
Good repetition	
Good naming	Normal
Poor naming	Anomic (MCA, angular gyrus)
Poor repetition	Conduction (MCA, arcuate fasciculus)
Poor Comprehension	
Good repetition	Transcortical sensory (PCA, parieto-occipital)
Poor repetition	Wernicke's (MCA, temporal)

Non-Fluent

Good Comprehension	
Good repetition	Transcortical Motor (ACA, prefrontal)
Poor repetition	Broca's (MCA, frontal lobe)
Poor Comprehension	
Good repetition	Mixed transcortical (ACA/PCA, watershed)
Poor repetition	Global (MCA, multilobar)

Other

Subcortical	Thalamus and basal ganglia
Alexia with agraphia	PCA, angular gyrus
Alexia without agraphia	PCA, medial-occipital and splenium of corpus callosum

ASIA Scale

A. Complete. No motor or sensory down to sacral level.

B. Sensory incomplete. No motor, some sensory below level and includes sacral segments S4–S5.

C. Motor incomplete. More than half of key muscles below neurological level are grade <3. Some sparing of sensory and/or motor in sacral segments S4, S5. Must have either (1) voluntary anal sphincter contraction or (2) motor sparing more than 3 levels below motor level.

D. Motor incomplete. More than half of key muscles below neurological level are grade ≥3. Some sparing of sensory and/or motor in sacral segments S4, S5. Must have either (1) voluntary anal sphincter contraction or (2) motor sparing more than 3 levels below motor level.

E. Normal (reflexes may be abnormal)

Level	Function	Muscle
C5	Elbow flexors	Biceps, Brachialis
C6	Wrist extensors	Extensor Carpi Radialis
C7	Elbow extensors	Triceps
C8	Finger flexors	Flexor Digitorum Profundus
T1	Small Finger Abductors	Abductor Digiti Minimi
L2	Hip flexors	Iliopsoas
L3	Knee extensors	Quadriceps
L4	Ankle dorsiflexors	Tibialis Anterior
L5	Long toe extensors	Extensor Hallucis Longus
S1	Ankle plantar flexors	Gastrocnemius

ASIA level is based on most caudal spinal segment with normal function based on motor for C5-T1, L2-S1 or sensory for all other levels. Motor level is defined by the lowest key muscle that has a grade ≥ 3 providing the level above is 5.
Determine zone of partial preservation: number of partially intact dermatomes and myotomes caudal to the neurological level.

(Adapted from International Standards for Neurological and Functional Classification of Spinal Cord Injury. Reprinted with permission of American Spinal Injury Association, Chicago, 2000).

II

Therapeutics

Modalities

Heat

vasodilation, ↓ pain, ↓ spasm, ↓ joint stiffness, ↑ ROM
↑ Metabolic rate, ↓ firing rate of muscle spindles
Superficial heat: hot packs
Paraffin: dip to coat extremity
Fluidotherapy: Hot air blown through particles
Infrared lamp: no contact with skin, local
Deep heat (Ultrasound) bone-soft-tissue interface
0.5–2.0 watts/cm2 x 5–10 min daily.
Phonophoresis: U/S + hydrocortisone, dexamethasone
Or 1% lidocaine (tendonitis) 1–2 MHz, 1–3 W/cm2
5–7 min
Contraindications to heat: acute inflammation, infection, trauma, bleeding, ischemia insensate skin, inability to respond to pain, malignancy, atrophic skin, edema, open wound.
Additional contraindications to ultrasound: fluid filled cavities, heart, brain, pacemakers, laminectomy site, thrombophlebitis, growing epiphyses, osteomyelitis, tumor, metal hardware and cement (hip prostheses)

Cold

Vasoconstriction, ↓ nerve conduction, ↓ edema & inflammation
Cold packs: use X 20–30 min
Ice message: analgesia in 7–10 min
Vapocoolant sprays: spray & stretch ethyl Cl or fluoromethane spasms, local skin anesthesia

Electrical current

Iontophoresis: direct current with lidocaine, hydrocortisone, dexamethasone
TENS: for pain, 30–60 min up to 8x/d

Contrast baths: alternate cold & warm baths—reflex hyperemia

Biofeedback: EMG, pressure, BP, respiratory, temp
Spinal Traction: cervical (manual, mechanical)
Restorative Manipulation: high velocity/low amplitude (thrust) at end ROM
Muscle energy techniques: isometric contraction, relaxation
Message & myofascial release
Accupuncture/accupressure: NIH accepted for control of pain and nausea

Strengthening

Strength gained in first few weeks of training is due to enhanced synchronization and recruitment of motor units. Muscle hypertrophy starts after 2–4 weeks.
Hypertrophy: repair of damaged muscle, ↑ capacity of oxidative metabolism

Isometric "same length"

Static muscular contraction without movement.
Best when near maximal and held for ~6 sec & repeated 5–10 times/day
Protects the joint from stress. Less inflammatory response.
Useful for limiting atrophy during immobilization. (i.e. cast)

Isotonic "same tension"

Theoretically, constant dynamic muscle contraction against same weight.
Realistically, tension does change through the range of motion of a joint.
Concentric: Loading of a muscle while it shortens. (lifting)
Eccentric: Loading of a muscle while it lengthens. (lowering)
May cause more soreness and hypertrophy

Isokinetic "same speed"

Maximal force through full range of motion with constant velocity.
Used for rehab of a particular joint and muscle with progressive torque i.e. throwing

Resistance band - "theraband": Resistance increases when stretched. Used in multiple planes for functional movements and sports activities.
Variable resistance (Cybex, Nautilus): Resistance is altered through the range using pulleys to match the actual capacity of a muscle.

Pylometric exercise: Fast concentric contractions after a weighted stretch. Jumping on and off different surfaces. Builds power and speed for sports.

Closed Kinetic Chain Exercise: Distal limb is anchored distally while multiple proximal joints move by agonist and antagonist movement i.e. squats, pushups, leg press, retrowalking, medicine ball.
More function based, sport-specific, multi-muscular, joint/ligament safer.

IV Heparin Weight based Normogram

Bolus 80 units/kg
25,000 units / 250 cc D5W @ 18 units/kg/hr
Check PTT 6 hours later and adjust:

PTT	
<36.5	Bolus 80 units/kg, ↑ 4 units/kg/hr
36.6–45.7	Bolus 80 units/kg, ↑ 2 units/kg/hr
45.8–70	No change
70.1–91.4	↓ 2 units/kg/hr
91.5	Hold for 1 hour, ↓ 3 units/kg/hr

Weight (kg)	50	60	70	80
Bolus 80u/kg	4000	4800	5600	6400
Units/hr	900	1080	1260	1440

Based on 25,000 units/250cc D5W concentration				
Drip cc/hr	9	11	12	14
2 units/kg/hr	1	1	1	1–2
3 units/kg/hr	1–2	2	2	2–3
4 units/kg/hr	2	2–3	3	3

Based on 25,000 units/500cc D5W concentration				
Drip cc/hr	18	22	25	29
2 units/kg/hr	2	2–3	3	3
3 units/kg/hr	3	3-4	4	5
4 units/kg/hr	4	5	5-6	6

After PTT therapeutic, start Coumadin 5mg QD and follow INR:
Daily for first 3–4 days to avoid over shoot
Give same dose for 2–3 days and check INR
Adjust dose and repeat same dose for 2–3 days and check INR
Try to limit blood draw to twice a week

(Adapted from Table 1, Raschke, etal. the Weight-Based Heparin dosing Normogram Compared with a "Standard Care" Normogram. Ann Intern Med. 1993; 119:874-881, with permission).

Orthoses

Shoes

Oxford depth (extra depth) inlay shoe
Med/Lat wedge, heel lift/wedge, longitudinal arch support, cushioned heel
Rocker bar, high toe box, metatarsal bar/pad, 1st/5th MT head relief, toe crest
Cast boot, Plastazote shoe (Neoprene)

UCBL: rigid plastic shoe insert, corrects pes planus/valgus
Heel cup: short insert, controls lateral calcaneal shift

AFO:

Posterior leaf spring (PLS): minimal ankle control, bends to PF/DF
Solid: good ankle control, rigid ankle, covers maleoli
Hinged: adjustable ankle hinge, DF/PF stops or assists
Spiral & Hemispiral – more expensive, minimal ankle control
Anterior tibial band – prevent buckling
T strap – varus or valgus correction

KAFO: Adds a knee hinge and thigh cuff
Uprights: Single or double upright metal
Locks: drop ring locks, spring loaded pull rod, pawl lock, fan lock
Craig-Scott: for paraplegics, pawl lock, bail release, shoe connected

HKAFO: Add pelvic band and hip joint

THKAFO: RGO (reciprocal gait orthosis) difficult to donn

Opponens: position weak thumb for function, C-bar, ± wrist control
Lumbrical bar: prevents MCP extension, anti "claw" position
Finger extension assist
Cock-up splint: volar wrist flexion control
Prehension orthoses: wrist or finger driven, passive
Universal splints: utensil holder
Resting hand splint: protective and prevents contractures
BFO: balanced forearm orthoses for proximal weakness
Collars: soft, rigid (Philadelphia, SOMI, halo)

TLSO: flex/ext control
Corsets: TLS, LS, SI
CTLSO: Milwaukee brace
TL: Jewett, Boston, CASH

Gait Aids

SC (straight cane): J handle, functional grip, curved top
NBQC (narrow based quad cane): 4 points, good for stairs
WBQC (wide based quad cane): 4 points, better stability
HW (hemi-walker): 1 handed for hemiplegics, wide based support

SW (standard walker): requires lifting, good balance, hand strength
RW (rolling walker): easier to use, no lifting
PW (platform walker): forearm support, minimal hand use, UE contractures
Rolling triceps walker: weight bearing on full arms, minimal hand use
Reciprocal walker: each side advances independently, B/L THR's
Reverse rollator: large RW, open in front, CP kids, promotes extension
Stair climbing walker: only for stair use, requires UE strength
AC (arm/axillary crutch): requires good balance, UE strength
Lofstrand crutch: utilizes forearms, can free hands to open doors

Gait Patterns

Walker

FWB: lift, place walker, advance 1st foot, advance 2nd foot past 1st foot
PWB: lift, place walker, advance affected foot, transfer weight to arms, advance unaffected foot

Crutches

4-point gait: R crutch, L foot, L crutch, R foot
3-point gait: both crutches with affected leg, then good leg
2-point gait: R crutch + L foot, L crutch + R foot
Swing-to gait: Advance crutches, lift weight & swing to level of crutches
Swing-through gait: Advance crutches, lift weight & swing beyond crutches

Cane

Use contralateral to affected side, i.e. R TKR, cane in left hand
One cane gait: cane + affected side, good side
Stairs: Up with the "good," down with the "bad"

Prosthetics—Lower Extremity

Toe: shoe filler
TMA/Lisfranc: molded socket, rigid plate
Chopart (calc, talus remain): plastic calf shell
Syme (calcaneal fat pad over maleoli) stump shell with SACH foot

Transtibial (BKA)

Foot

SACH (solid ankle, cushion heel) cheap, simple
Single axis vs. multi-axis (SAFE, endolite) - allows inversion/eversion
Energy storing: Seattle (light), STEN, Carbon copy, flex foot – expensive

Shank

Endoskeletal: pylon covered with foam, cosmetic, adjustable, wears easily
Exoskeleton: rigid shell, non-adjustable, durable

Socket

Custom molded, rigid outer, flexible inner, PTB (patellar tendon bearing)

Suspension

Supracondylar cuff ± fork strap & waist belt,
Supracondylar/suprapatellar brim, sleeve (neoprene, silicone)
ICEROSS: roll-on silicone sleeve with pin locking into socket
Alpha liner: low resistance roll-on silicone sleeve, no pin.

Transfemoral (AKA)

Knee

Single axis, polycentric axis (4 bar)
Friction: constant, variable (sliding, hydraulic, pneumatic)
Manual lock
Mauch Swing & stance: weight activated friction brake
Extension aids: internal or external

Socket

Quadralateral (old), Ischial Containment (CAT-CAM, narrow ML)

Suspension

Total suction suspension – one-way valve
Silesien belt, TES (total elastic suspension) belt, pelvic band & hip joint

Amputation Rehabilitation

Precautions: Sensory loss, stump wound, fall & balance, avoid trauma to residual limb, cardiac parameters if vascular insufficiency (Max HR: 220 – age x 70%) and avoid valsalva & excessive UE isometrics.

Posterior extension splint worn at all times when not in therapy. Extension board on wheelchair, ace wrap, compression stocking or rigid dressing at all times except for inspection and limb care.

PT: A/AAROM LE's. Isotonic PRE's.
Static stretching: iliopsoas, gluts, quads, hams, gastocs.
Encourage prone lying/knee and hip extension in bed.
Skin care/stump inspection, compressive dressing and training.
Prosthetic training & parts management.
Improve balance/coordination in static/dynamic ranges with and without prosthesis,
Bed mobility and transfer training,
Wheelchair mobility and parts management.
Progressive prosthetic ambulation training, community ambulation training (stairs, ramps, curbs), fall recovery techniques, safety training.
Scar mobilization/stump massage, desensitization, HEP.

OT: ADLs & Adaptive equipment eval,
Teach sensory precautions, energy conservation.
Improve UE coordination, functional gross grasp strength, pinch strength. A/AAROM, isotonic PRE's, static stretching.
Improve sitting/standing balance in static/dynamic ranges with ADL's. Stump care, prosthetic care and management, kitchen eval, safety training. HEP.

TR: Improve standing balance/tolerance/endurance. Improve coordination. UE dexterity, strength. ↑ Prosthetic acceptance & use during activities.

Myofascial Trigger Point Treatment

Myofascial Pain Syndrome: A regional pain complaint with pain or altered sensation in an expected distribution of referred pain from a trigger point with a taut band, point tenderness in 1 spot and some restriction of ROM. May also have reproduction of pain upon palpation of tender spot, a local twitch response and relief of pain by stretch or injection.

Tender spots: Small localized tender points or taut bands of muscle fibers within muscle, fascia, tendons, ligaments, periosteum, & pericapsular areas.
Trigger points: Point which "triggers" pain in another area
Referred pain: Pain caused by distant trigger point
Taut band: Palpable groups of involuntary contracting muscle fibers
Causes: posture, stress, sprains, overuse, systemic disease
Common sites:
Upper: suboccipital, paraspinals, levator scapulae, supraspinatus, infraspinatus, rhomboids, wrist extensors, traps
Lower: Sacrospinatus, quadratus lumborum, gluteal, TFL, vastus medialis, gastrocnemius and soleus.

Vapocoolant spray (ethyl chloride): inhibit pain & spinal stretch reflex
Aspirate syringe, inject 0.1–0.3cc at a time up to 3cc in 1 area
Injection: 25-gauge needle, 1.5–3.5 inch (1% lidocaine)
Pre-injection block: infiltrate area proximal to taut band
TP Injection: Needle and infiltration of taut band and fibrotic core
Post-injection: rest, short course NSAIDs, PT (heat, TENS, spray & stretch)

Spray & stretch: Fluorimethane or ethyl chloride in direction of muscle fibers while passively stretching (30 seconds). Follow with hot pack and slow active ROM through full range. Repeat 5 times.

Fibromyalgia: diffuse and generalized tender points involving bilateral and symmetrical muscle and non-muscle tissue. There are no areas of referred pain and no taut bands. Do not respond to trigger point injection
Typically involves 11 of 18 points (ACR). Controversy exists over the existence of the diagnosis.

III

Specific Disorders

Deep Vein Thrombosis

Virchow's Triad: Venous stasis, endothelial injury, coagulopathy
Usually forms in distal LE veins and extends proximally.
Becomes significant at popliteal fossa when risk of embolization increases.
Organization of a mature thrombus takes 7–10 days.
Standard of treatment on rehab is to limit involved LE therapy (muscle contraction) for 72 hours after therapeutic anticoagulation. Can then follow with full therapy program.

Risk factors: General anesthesia, immobility, surgery, trauma, obesity, hypotension, DM, stasis dermatitis, CHF, prior DVT, age, infection, malignancy.

Physical signs: LE swelling, popliteal/calf tenderness & erythema, ↑ girth, Homan's sign, palpable cord (many DVT's are asymptomatic)

Duplex Doppler Ultrasound (proximal > calf)
Impedence Plethysmography
Venography

Treatment: If in popliteal vein or above → anticoagulate
(Superficial femoral vein DVT should be treated)
IV Heparin, Lovenox (1mg/kg BID), IVC filter (if ↑ bleeding risk)
Usually switch to Coumadin and continue for 6 wks–6 months

Prophylaxis
Intermittent pneumatic leg compression (venodynes)
Compression stockings (teds) ASA
Coumadin (INR 2.0–2.5) SQ heparin
Lovenox (Enoxaparin) 40 mg qd (THR), 30 mg bid (TKR, ortho surg, SCI, cancer surgery, trauma)

Suspect PE: malaise, fever, SOB, chest pain, tachycardia, tachypnea
EKG: S1, P3, T3, ABG: A-a gradient $[(713 \times F_iO_2) - (PaCO2/0.8)] - P_aO_2$
V/Q scan, CT Angiogram, Pulmonary angiogram

Complex Regional Pain Syndrome

Reflex Sympathetic Dystrophy • Causalgia
Shoulder-hand syndrome • Sympathalgia • Sudeck's atrophy

Chronic painful condition of a limb (UE>LE), etiology unkown.
Caused by sympathetic instability
Painful impairment of the shoulder & hand edema
10–15% of all patients with hemiplegia and painful shoulder
Affects distal region of limb

CRPS Type 1	(RSD) occurs after noxious event, i.e., trauma, surgery, radicolopathy, MI, Visceral disease, CNS lesion (CVA), Fracture
CRPS Type 2	(Causalgia) occurs after nerve injury
Stage 1	(weeks to 6 months), Pain, ↑ blood flow, pitting edema, redness, warmth, hyperhydrosis (sweating), ↓ ROM, hyperesthetic skin early osteoporosis (not seen on x-ray)
Stage 2	(3 to 6 months later), ↑ pain, ↓ blood flow, ↓ edema, coldness brawny edema, hyperhydrosis, further ↓ ROM Xrays- patchy localized osteoporosis, periarticular thickening
Stage 3	(Persists for months), ↓ pain, skin smooth, glossy, dry, cool irreversible atrophic muscle & soft tissue, severe ↓ ROM x-rays – extensive osteoporosis, coarse hair and ridged nails

Dx: 3-phase bone scan (pooling phase most sensitive)

Tx: Medrol pack, NSAIDs, calcitonin, neurontin, epidural (LE)
Desensitization: isotoner gloves, contrast baths, U/S, paraffin, TENS, acupuncture
Edema control: Elevation, retrograde message, compression devices
Fluoroscopic sympathetic block

Regional IV Bier block (guanethidine, methylprednisolone + lidocaine, phenoxybenzamine),
Surgical sympathectomy
Percutaneous electrical stim, dorsal column stim, deep brain stim

Guillain-Barré Syndrome

Acute Inflammatory Demyelinating Polyneuropathy

Acquired, symmetrical polyneuropathy
Lower extremities usually affected 1st
Usually begins with distal paresthesias, then ascending weakness
Weakness progresses over days to weeks, areflexia
Can cause total quadraparesis and respiratory failure
Facial and oropharyngeal muscles often involved
Extraocular muscles and sphincters usually spared
Mild sensory symptoms, autonomic dysfunction (orthostatics)
Recovery begins 2–4 weeks after progression ceases
CSF - ↑ protein, <10 WBC's/mm3

EMG: Prolonged or absent F,H, ↓ motor CV, temporal dispersion, ↑ DL
Segmental demyelination, motor > sensory
↓ Prognosis: Needle EMG with spontaneous activity, CMAP <10% (indicates axonal loss)

Tx: Plasmaphoresis,
Monitor Vital capacity (<1 Liter consider ventilation)

Rehab:
Early: ROM exercises, positioning. Static splints
Non-fatiguing strengthening
Later: Tilt table, standing frame, parallel bars
90–95% complete recovery

CIDP: Chronic inflammatory demyelinating polyneuropathy
Chronic form with relapses and exacerbations
Treat relapses with steroids

Miller-Fisher variant: Ataxia, ophthalmoplegia, ↓ reflexes

Multiple Sclerosis

Exact etiology unknown
Demyelination of brain and spinal cord
Affects gait, coordination, bladder, sexual function
Incidence ↑ with Northern latitude, 70% female
CSF: ↑γ-globulin, oligoclonal bands (+ in 90%)
MRI: Plaques in white matter (periventricular) 3–4 lesions >3mm
Evoked potentials: abnormalities on VEP, BAEP, SSEP

Presenting symptoms: Weakness, paresthesias, gait difficulty, optic neuritis, diplopia,
ataxia, poor nutrition, vertigo

Common signs and symptoms: *(in decreasing order of prevalence)*
Paresthesias, weakness, abnormal reflexes, cerebellar signs, spasticity, fatigue, ↓ RAM, heat intolerance, nystagmus, intellectual loss, impotence, Lhermitte's sign, pain, depression, muscle wasting, dementia, facial weakness, unilateral hearing loss, epilepsy, visual loss, trigeminal neuralgia

Optic neuritis: unilateral eye pain, central scotoma
Pain: 50% of pts, chronic dysesthetic extremity, back pain, leg cramps
Severe disability: 10% at 5 years, 25% at 10 years, 50% at 18 years
Tx: IV Steroids (decrease length and severity of acute exacerbations)
Interferon β (decreases exacerbation rates) Avonex Qwk, Betaseron TIW
Copaxone (glatiramer) 20mg SC qd
Weakness: general conditioning, avoid ↑ fatigue & body temperature
Air-resistance bikes, cool pools, UE ergometer, light weight resistance
Fatigue: Pemoline (18.75mg/d), symmetrel 200–300mg/d
Cognitive: memory, conceptual, abstraction, apathy, slowness, depression
Neurogenic bladder (hyperreflexia, DESD) ✓ PVR, UDS
Neurogenic bowel: ↑ fiber, bulk former, stool softeners, supp, laxatives
Spasticity: See spasticity section
Sexual function: counseling, ED: Viagra, injections, implants
Ataxia: Splinting, Meds have minimal affect - Clonazepam, primidone, INH
Painful paresthesias: Neurontin

Kurtzke Disability Status Scale

0	Normal exam
1	No disability, minimal signs (ie babinski)
2	Minimal disability
3	Moderate disability, fully ambulatory
4	Relatively severe disability, fully ambulatory Self sufficient, up & about 12 hr/d
5	Severe disability, unable to work full day without provisions maximal motor function, walking unaided several blocks
6	Ambulate with AD
7	Restricted to WC, self-propel, transfer independently
8	Restricted to bed, effective use of arms
9	Bedridden
10	Death

Spasm Frequency Score

0	No spasms
1	Mild spasm with stimulation
2	Infrequent, full spasm, <1/hour
3	Spasm >1/hour
4	Spasms 10+/hour, or continuous contraction

Movement Disorders

Idiopathic:	Secondary
Parkinson's disease	Birth injury
Progressive supranuclear palsy	Chorea Gravidarum
Multiple system atrophy (Shy-Drager)	Neuroleptic meds
Corticobasal degeneration	Head injury
Most dystonias	Cerebral infarct/hemorrhage
Blepharospasm	Anoxia
Meige's disease	Carbon Monoxide poisoning
Gilles de la Tourette's syndrome	Manganese poisoning
Genetic:	Mercury poisoning
Huntington's disease	Basal Ganglia tumor
Wilson's disease	Liver disease
Some dystonias	Oral contraceptives
Inherited ataxias	Thyroid disease
Metabolic defects	Hypoparathyroidism
Ataxia Telangiectasia	Alcohol
Olivopontocerebellar degeneration	Sydenham's chorea
Friedreich's ataxia	von Economo's encephalitis
Familiar nonprogressive chorea	
Essential tremor	

Clinical features of Parkinson's disease

Rigidity	Bradykinesia, Hypokinesia
Resting/postural tremor	Loss of postural reflexes
Akathisia (inability to sit still)	Dementia
Autonomic dysfunction	Dysarthria, dysphasia
Festinating gait	Masked fascies
Dystonia, Flexed posture	Freezing of motor activity

Medications and common side effects

Levodopa	Nausea, ↓ BP, arrythmias, hallucinations/ psychosis
Deprenyl	Cardiac toxic, hallucinations (potentiates L-dopa)
Amantadine	Hallucinations, insomnia, anxiety, edema, headache
Dopa agonists	Hallucinations, vivid dreams, psychosis, paranoia
Anticholinergics	↓ memory, confusion, urinary retention, vision blurred

Parkinson's Disease Therapy Orders

PT:

A/AA/P ROM, prevent contractures
Stretch: spine, pectoralis, individual tight muscles that decrease function.
Isometric strengthening of quads, gluts.
Back flexion/extension exercise, pelvic tilt
Relaxation techniques to ↓ rigidity, slow rhythmic rotational movements,
Proper sitting & postural control, mat activities, tilt table if needed,
Bed mobility, transfer training, rocking to elevate from chair,
Stationary bike for reciprocal training, PNF, biofeedback,
NDT training to facilitate slow movement.
Training in rhythmic pattern to music to auditory cues.
Standing balance in parallel bars with weight shifting.
Progressive ambulation training, proper heel-toe gait training, step over blocks, feet 12–15" apart, arm swinging.
Assistive devices, cardiac fitness training. Frequent rests,
Frankel's exercises for ataxia. Family training and HEP.

OT:

A/AA/P ROM UE's and stretching of tight muscles.
Fine motor coordination skills, ADL eval & training,
Hand cycling for reciprocal movements, rocking chair to help mobilization, transfer training, safety skills, handwriting skills,
Adaptive devices with Velcro closures, raised toilet seat, grab bars,
Eating utensils, built up handles, key holders, etc.
Positioning & posture training, family training & HEP.

ST:

Diaphragmatic breathing, swallowing eval & training with icing, supraglottal swallow, vibration, compensatory chin tuck.
Hypokinetic dysarthria training, deep breathing exercises, facial, oral & lingual muscle training and coordination.

TR:

Activities to promote posture, coordination, standing endurance.

Spinal Cord Injury

Incidence: 30–60 /mil Prevalence: 700–900/mil M:F=4:1
C1-T12 UMN injury: ↑ reflexes, clonus, babinski, DESD
LMN at level of injury
L1-L2: Conus Medularis (mixed UMN & LMN)
L3-S5: LMN injury: ↓ reflexes, flaccid weakness, atrophy
Spinal shock: Lack of descending facilitation. Flaccid days-weeks

C2-C4:	high quad, vent dependant, trach, power wc (sip & puff) Phrenic n. pacing, assist for all ADL, 24° care, ECU
C5:	assist ADL, universal cuff, power wc
C6:	tenodesis splint, modified Ind., cathing, SB tx, manual wc Drive modified van
C7-C8:	Independent transfer without SB
T1-T12:	truncal stability, improved cough, autonomic dysreflexia >T6
Lumbar:	May ambulate with AFO, KAFO, ↑ energy demand

Anterior cord syndrome – variable loss of motor, pinprick, temp.
Sparing of priopriocеption, anterior spinal artery (Adamkevitz)
Central cord syndrome – cervical hyper-extension injury, paresis UE>LE
Bladder, bowel, sexual varies
Brown-Sequard syndrome – hemi-section, ipsilateral motor, proprioception
Contralateral pinprick, temp, good prognosis
Conus Medularis/Cauda Equina – areflexic bladder,bowel, flaccid paralysis

Problems (see each section for details)

- Bladder
- Bowel
- Contractures
- Spasticity
- Pressure ulcers
- Neuropathic pain
- DVT ppx
- Osteoporosis
- Syringomyelia
- Autonomic dysfunction
- Sexual dysfunction
- Heterotopic Ossification
- Psychological adaptation
- Depression
- Environmental modification
- Vocational/Avocational
- Wheelchair and equipment
- SMA syndrome

Bladder Management

Parasympathetic (chol) – Pelvic n. (S-234) detruser contraction emptying
Sympathetic (α) hypogastric n. (T10-L2) internal sphincter storage
Somatic – Pudendal n. (S-234) external sphincter storage

Need UDS to test dysfunction, but can predict by location

UMN Bladder

Supraspinal (above pontine micturition center)
    Hyper-reflexia, detruser instability, low volumes, high pressures, ↓ compliance, leaking (from bladder spasms), incontinence
Suprasacral (between pons and sacral micturition center)
    DESD (detruser external sphincter dysenergia)
    As above with sphincter contracting at same time as voiding

Treatment:

Anticholinergics Ditropan 5mg bid (XL qd), Detrol 1–2mg bid,
  SE: dry mouth, blurry vision, n/v, sedation, tachy, retention, constipation
Alpha blockers for ↑ sphincter tone Hytrin, Cardura, Flomax, Minipress
  SE: hypotension, sedation, headaches, syncope, retrograde ejaculation
    Hyoscyamine .125–.250mg tid-qid, Imipramine (25mg tid)
    Intermittent catheterization, suprapubic tapping
    Bladder augmentation (↑ capacity) with catheterization
    Sphincterotomy with condom cath in males
    Ileal conduit – requires catheterization through stoma

LMN bladder

Infrasacral (conus, cauda equina, peripheral nerves)
    Hypotonic detruser and/or sphincter, retention
    Overflow incontinence
Mixed UMN & LMN (sacral, conus, peripheral neuropathy, MS)
Treatment: condom catheter, foley, intermittent catheterization
    Evacuation with crede, valsalva (chol agonists are ineffective)

Intermittent catheterization: Q4-6 hours, volumes should be <400–500cc
    ↓ fluid intake in evening, try to avoid night time catheterization
Indwelling catheter: Change every 4 weeks (stones, prostatitis, stricture)
    Cystoscopy q2 years for transitional and squamous cell carcinoma

Bowel Management

Auerbach's plexus – myenteric, between muscle layers - primarily motor
Meissner's plexus – submucosal, primarily sensory
Parasympathetic (chol) – vagus & pelvic n. – gut stimulation
Sympathetic – hypogastric n. (T10-L2) – gut relaxation
Somatic – pudendal n. (S-234) ext sphincter and pelvic floor muscles

UMN bowel

Ext sphincter cannot relax with ↑ tone, spastic pelvic floor muscles.
Intrinsic reflexes and peristalsis intact.
Medications, stimulation and timed evacuation most helpful.

LMN bowel

Areflexic bowel, slow propulsion, constipation & impaction
Neurogenic fecal incontinence is not common
Anal tone still present 2° reflexive internal sphincter
Manual disimpaction and bulking agents most helpful.

Attempt timed QOD evacuation.
Minimize TCA, narcotics which ↓ bowel motility
Diet with adequate fluid, fiber, prune juice, dairy
Whole grain bread, bran cereal, wheat germ, fruits & vegetables
Metamucil / Citrocal
Start with Colace 100mg TID & Sennekot 1–2tabs QHS
Dulcolax supp Qam 20min after breakfast
Then add Dulcolax tabs, fleets enemas, therevac PRN
Mg citrate, high colonic enemas, manual disimpaction
Gastrocolic reflex – time evacuation 1 hour after breakfast
Rectocolic reflex – digital stimulation/suppository
Ileostomy or colostomy in refractory dysmotility
Partial ext sphincter myotomy for dyssenergia

Pressure Ulcers

Risk factors: immobility, ↓ nutrition, spasticity, contractures, positioning, incontinence, dementia, pressure, shearing, friction

Common sites: Sacrum, coccyx, ischial tuberosity, greater trochanter, Occiput, scapulae, heels

Prevention: change position Q2 hours, bunny boots, pillows, multipodas boots, proper wheelchair cushion and mattress.
Skin care – triple care nursing care, aloe vesta, curity

Stage I – non-blanching erythema
Relieve pressure, gauze, transparency film (opsite, tegaderm)

Stage II – erosion through epidermis into dermis, blister/abrasion
Specialty (primapore, band-aid, telfa, covaderm)

Stage III – through subcutaneous tissue, i.e. fat
Hydrocolloid (duoderm, comfeel)
Mild-mod exudates: Gels (solosite, curasol sheets)

Stage IV – extension to fascia, muscle, bone
Hydrocolloid & gels
Heavy exudates: alginates (sorbsan), foams (allevyn, polymem)

Debridement: enzymatic, surgical, wet→dry
Nutrition: Protein intake 1–1.25g/kg, Vit C 500mg bid, Zn (if ↓)
Treat anemia, Fe, Folate, B12 deficiency

Static overlays (polyurethane foam, gel-filled, air-filled, water filled)
Dynamic overlays, alternating pressure-point mattress, rolling mattress
Air-fluidized bed (clinitron) good for drying heavy exudates
Low air-loss bed (Alamo, Kin-air)
Skin graft, skin flap, myocutaneous flap, free flap (grade III or IV)
Chair cushions: Roho (air cells), Jay2 (gel)

Contractures

Fixed ↓ ROM 2° collagen deposition in response to injury
Athrogenic: intrinsic derangement, OA, Fx
Soft tissue: shortened tendons, ligaments, skin
Myogenic: MDA, spasticity, immobility, pain, position.

Common sites:

Ankle plantarflexion, knee flexion, hip flexion
Elbow flexion, shoulder adduction/internal rotation
Muscles that cross 2 joints: gastroc, TFL, hamstring, biceps.

Prevention:

Early mobilization, ROM, positioning and braces/splints.
Supine position, shoulders in abduction, elbows in extension
AFO or multipodas boots.
Wheelchairs should have arms rests or lapboard.

Treatment:

Treat spasticity, pain and adjust positioning.
Stretch with heat/ultrasound, terminal sustained stretch.
Serial casting Q3–5 days
Dynamic splinting: esp. knee extension and ankle DF aids.
Surgery: joint manipulation, tendon release/lengthening

Functional contractures:

C6-C7 quadriplegia, allow MCP, PIP, DIP to contract ~20°
Use a wrist driven tenodesis orthosis for ↑ function.

Autonomic Dysfunction

Dysfunction of sympathetic and parasympathetic tone causes
Orthostatic hypotension, altered temperature regulation, ↓ sweating, ↓ GI motility, sexual dysfunction

Treatment of hypotension: volume expanders
NaCl tablets
Florinef 0.1mg qd *(SE: htn, chf, ↓ K+ alkalosis, edema ↓ Na+)*
Ephedrine 25mg bid *(SE: tachy, arrhythmia, palps, ha)*
Midodrine 2.5mg tid *(SE: ha, paresthesias, dysuria, pruritis)*
Compression stockings, abdominal binders

Autonomic Dysreflexia

Occurs in SCI above T6 2° loss of autonomic tone
Hypertension, brady or tachycardia, sweating, flushing (above level), pallor (below level), headache, nasal congestion, anxiety.

Causes: Bladder distention, impaction, UTI, skin ulcers, ingrown toe nail, tight clothing, fractures, stones, intra-abdominal pathology, cystoscopy/colonoscopy, HO, childbirth
Severe uncontrolled htn may cause: confusion, visual disturbance, LOC, encephalopathy, intracerebral hemorrhage, Sz, EKG changes, Afib, MI

Treatment: Sit up, remove all potential noxious stimuli: Cath/change foley, disimpact with lidocaine jelly, check skin, treat UTI
If BP still elevated, then . . .
Sublingual: Nifedipine 10mg Topical: Nitropaste
IV: phentolamine 5–10mg, diazoxide 100–250mg, Hydralazine 10mg (slow)
Pentolinium 5–10mg, MethylDopa 250mg (slow)

Chronic Recurrent Dysreflexia (PO):
Phenoxybenzamine 30–60mg bid, Clonidine 0.1–0.2mg tid or patch 0.1–0.3,
Prazosin 1–2mg bid, Mecamylamine 5mg tid,
Pentolinium 20–40mg qid Methyldopa 250mg qid

Spasticity

Velocity dependant resistance to passive movement
Part of the Upper Motor Neuron Syndrome
Spasticity may be functional (evaluate carefully before treating)
Treatment indications: Pain, deformities, poor positioning for hygiene, prevent & treat pressure ulcers, improve gait and transfers

Treatment

Identify stimuli, i.e. UTI, stones, impaction, HO, ulcers
Position: partially recumbant, bracing, ↑ sensory information
Modalities: cold, TENS may be useful (caution with insensate)
PT: Daily terminal sustained stretch

Meds:

Baclofen (GABA analogue) 2.5mg bid (max 160mg/d)
(SE: sedation, weakness, fatigue, n/v, dizzy, sz, paresthesias)
Diazepam (GABA facilitation) 2.5mg bid (max 60mg/d)
(SE: sedation, weakness, depression, ataxia, ↓ memory)
Clonidine (central α-2 agonist) 0.1mg bid or 0.1mg patch
(SE: sedation, weakness, dry mouth, constipation, ↓ BP)
Tizanidine (central α-2 agonist) 2mg bid (max 36mg/d)
(SE: same as Clonidine + hepatic toxicity (LFTs)
Dantrolene (inhibits Ca2+ release) 25mg qd (max 400mg/d)
(SE: sedation, weakness, dizzy, paresthesias, n/v/d, hepatic toxicity)
(Tizanidine & Dantrolene: ✓ LFT's month 1,3,6 then yearly)

Phenol Nerve blocks (chemolysis): Try temporary block with lidocaine first to test usefulness
Blocks motor distribution and/or sensory to ↓ afferent information.
Duration of effect 3–9 months or longer.
(SE: paresthesias)

Botulinum Toxin (inhibits acetylcholine release): Duration 1–6 months.
Max 360–400 units per visit to avoid antibodies.

Baclofen pump: Delivers concentrated dose to intrathecal space.
Fill pump through abdomen every 1–3months.

Surgery: selective dorsal rhizotomy, spares motor, ↓ afferent input

Heterotopic Ossification

AKA: ectopic ossification, myositis ossificans

New bone formation within soft tissue occurring around joints.
Lesions are extra-articular
May be a genetic predisposition.
Affects patients with immobility and SCI. (10–20%)
Other risk factors: THR, burns, TBI
Ankylosis may occur in advanced cases.
Usually occurs within several months post injury
Hips and knees most common
Erythema, pain and edema, ↓ ROM, ↑ spasms, fevers

Diagnosis: ↑ alk phos, correlates with disease activity
Calcium may be elevated
radiographs: may not show early disease
3 phase bone scan: Shows areas of new bone formation (phase 1 & 2)
CT: May be used for planning surgical extraction

Treatment:

PT, maintain gentle ROM, ↓ pain
Etidronate (Didronel) 300mg IV qd x 3d, then 20mg/kg/d x 6 months *(SE: n/v/d)*
NSAIDS: May be of benefit. Indocin 25mg tid

Surgery: Failed therapy and medical management with significant joint contracture, poor positioning for hygiene and care, ↑ spasticity
Extraction is to restore movement.
Must wait up to 2 years when bone is mature and disease is inactive

Prophylactic Radiation therapy: 600–750 rads daily after surgical removal.

Sexual Dysfunction

Complex interaction of vascular, endocrine, CNS and PNS
4 stages: Arousal, Plateau, Orgasm, Resolution

Somatic - pudendal n. (S-234) sensory from penis, scrotum
Parasympathetic – pelvic n. (S-234) reflexic erection (tactile)
Sympathetic – hypogastric n. (T10-L2) – psychogenic erection & ejaculation

In SCI:

Erections are more successful with incomplete lesions
Ejaculation in 32% of incomplete UMN, 2% of complete UMN
Retrograde ejaculation is common

Meds:

Sildenafil (Viagra) type 5 phosphodiesterase inhibitor, 60min before sex
Most effective in patients with reflexic erections. 50–100mg PO
(SE: headache, flushing, visual disturbance, Avoid in cardiac disease)

Intracavernosal injection:

Alprostadil (Caverject), Phentolamine, papaverine
(SE: priapism, pain, penile fibrosis)

Penile Vacuum Devices:

Negative pressure chamber with rubber band (remove after 30min max)

Penile implants:

Simple malleable prosthesis, easiest to use, cosmetic problem
Hydraulic prosthesis: prone to mechanical failure

Fertility: rectal electroejaculation and penile vibroejaculation are used to harvest semen. Better success with incomplete SCI lesions.

Female lubrication: Artificial lubrication often necessary.

Deconditioning

Immobilization with reduced capacity of multiple systems.

Contracture: (see section) Treat: Daily terminal sustained stretching

Muscle Weakness and Atrophy:

With complete immobility, there is a 10–20% ↓ in isometric strength per week or 1–3% per day. Treat: voluntary contraction or electrical stimulation.

Osteoporosis:

Lack of weight bearing, hypercalciuria.
Cancellous bone resorption at metaphysis & epiphysis and later at diaphysis
Bone density is reduced 40–45% at 12 weeks of immobility.
Treat: standing exercise, standing frame, tilt table

Orthostatic hypotension:

Loss of ability to regulate BP 2° loss of autonomic tone
Treat: early mobilization, LE strengthening, abdominal strengthening
Tilt table, elastic stockings, abdominal binder

Cardiac deconditioning:

↑ resting HR (1/2 beat/d x 4 weeks)
↓ resting SV (15% after 2 weeks)
↓ cardiac size (11%) & ↓ LVEDV
↑ HR response to exercise
↓ circulating blood volume
↓ CO & ↓ VO_2 max (with exercise)

Respiratory:

↓ TV, VC, minute volume, ↓ diaphragm movement, atelectasis, pneumonia
Treat: chest PT, incentive spirometer, positioning, assisted cough

Skin: Ulcers, edema, bursitis. Treat: positioning, relieve pressure
GI: ↓ appetite, intestinal atrophy, constipation. Treat: bowel program
GU: diuresis, electrolyte imbalance, UTI, stones. Treat: fluids, position
Metabolic: ↓ lean mass, ↑ fat, hypercalcemia
Endocrine: glucose intolerance, altered hormone response

Dysphasia

Oral

Lip closure, lingual control, mastication & salivation
Dysfunction: Drooling, pocketing, repeat attempts, head tilt

Pharyngeal

Elevation of tongue, palate and larynx
Folding of epiglottis, vocal adduction, coordinated pharyngeal motility
Dysfunction: regurgitation, food sticking, cough, choke, wet voice

Esophageal

Coordinated peristalsis, LES relaxation, Cricopharyngeal contraction
Dysfunction: Food sticking, heartburn

Videofluoroscopy (modified barium swallow)
Dry swallow, thin liquid barium, thick liquid barium, solid barium cookie
Evaluate for penetration/aspiration, pooling in piriformis sinus & valleculae

FEESST (fiberoptic endoscopic)
Direct visualization of anatomy. Premature spillage, laryngeal penetration, tracheal aspiration, pharyngeal residue

Ultrasound
Good soft tissue delineation, but limited area, artifacts, missed aspiration

Complications of dysphasia: malnutrition, pneumonia

Treatment: (may include)

Dysphasia diet: pureed, semisolid, solid
Thickening agents, avoid thin liquids
Exercises: Lip, tongue & jaw strengthening, ROM, coordination
Strengthening & coordinating cough, vocal cord adduction
Thermal stimulation: ↑ speed of swallow
Compensatory: chin tuck, turn & tilt head, repeat swallow, alternate textures

Motor Neuron Disease

Upper Motor Neuron Disease

Primary lateral sclerosis
Tropical spastic paraparesis
Lathyrism
Epidemic spastic paraparesis
Familial spastic paraplegia

Upper and Lower Motor Neuron

ALS
Groote Eylandt
Juvenile inclusion body ALS
Western Pacific ALS (Parkinsonism Dementia Complex)
Familial ALS
Postencephalitic ALS
Lower Motor Neuron

Lower Motor Neuron Disease

Spinal Muscular Atrophy, Type I–V

I.	Acute Infantile SMA (Acute Werdnig-Hoffman)	AR
II.	Chronic Infantile SMA (Chronic Werdnig-Hoffman)	AR
III.	Juvenile & Adult proximal SMA (Kugelberg-Welander)	AR
IV.	Juvenile Dominant Proximal Hereditary Motor Neuropathy	AD
V.	Adult Dominant Proximal Hereditary Motor Neuropathy	AD

Childhood Bulbar (Fazio-Londe & Brown-Vialetto-van Laere)	AR
Distal SMA	AD
Scapuloperoneal muscular atrophy	AD/AR
Chronic bulbospinal muscular atrophy of Late Onset	XLR
Monomelic (segmental) SMA	
Monoclonal gammopathy	
Cancer	
Polio & post-polio syndrome	

Tests: EMG, muscle bx, SPEP, αAchR, HTLV-1, HIV, αGM1 & αGD_{1a}, Genetic testing

Problems: pain in acute polio, muscle tightening & contractures, spasticity, deformity, scoliosis, weakness, respiratory failure, dysphagia.

Neuropathy

	Seddon	Sunderland
Neurapraxia:	1st °	Focal conduction block, myelin injury
Axonotmesis:	2nd °	Axonal damage, Wallerian degeneration, intact sheaths
Neurotmesis:	3rd °	Injury to axon & endoneurium
	4th °	Injury to axon, endoneurium & perineurium
	5th °	Injury to all structures (transection)

Hereditary Peripheral neuropathies
CMT (HMSN type I & II)
Dejerine-Sottas (HMSN type III)
Refsum's (HMSN type IV)
Spinocerebellar degeneration (HMSN type V)
Optic atrophy (HMSN type VI)
Retinitis pigmentosa (HMSN type VII)
Friedreich's Ataxia
Pressure-sensitive hereditary neuropathy
Acute intermittent porphyria
Familial amyloid neuropathy
Fabry's disease
Hereditary sensory neuropathy
Giant axonal neuropathy
Lipoprotein neuropathy
Roussy-Levy syndrome
Riley-Day syndrome
Pelizaeus-Merzbacher
Metachromatic leukodystrophy
Krabbe's leukodystrophy
Tangier disease

Toxic Neuropathy
Amiodirone Dapsone
Corticosteroids
Disulfiram Heroin
Hydralazine INH
LSD Misonidazole
Nitrofurantoin Vit B6
Tetanus Thalidomide
Chloramphenicol
Cisplatin Vincristine

Heavy Metals
Antimony, Arsenic
Gold, Lead, Mercury
Thallium

Organic compounds
Ethyl alcohol
Acrylamide
Carbon Disulfide
Ethylene oxide
Methylbutyl ketone

Neuropathy associated diseases

Etoh	Amyloid	Gammopathy
Liver disease	COPD	Cryoglobinemia
Diabetes	Giant cell arteritis	Gout
Hypothyroidism	Necrotizing angiopathy	Malignancy

Idiopathic Neuropathy
Brachial neuritis (Parsonage-Turner)
Chronic inflammatory polyradiculopathy
Chronic relapsing polyneuropathy
Fisher syndrome
Guillian-Barre syndrome/CIDP
Steroid responsive polyneuropathy

Nutritional Deficiency Neuropathy
B_1, B_2, B_6, B_{12}

Infectious etiology
CMV, HIV, Diphtheria, Herpes, Leprosy, Rabies

Types of Diabetic Neuropathy
- Diffuse Neuropathy
- Distal symmetric sensorimotor polyneuropathy
- Autonomic neuropathy
  - Psuedomotor neuropathy
  - Cardiovascular autonomic neuropathy
  - Gastrointestinal neuropathy
  - Genitourinary neuropathy
- Symmetric proximal lower limb neuropathy

Focal Neuropathy
- Cranial mononeuropathy
- Radiculopathy/Plexopathy
- Entrapment neuropathy

Mononeuritis Multiplex

Multiple nerve infarcts due to vasculitis (polyarteritis nodosa, RA, SLE, Lyme, Sjögrens, cryoglobulinemia, temporal arteritis, scleroderma, sarcoid, leprosy, acute Hep A, AIDS) Diabetes with multiple compression sites.

Myopathy

Muscular Dystrophies

Duchenne	XLR	3–5	↓ amb, falls, Gowers'
Becker's	XLR	10–15	less severe than DMD
Fascioscapulohumeral	AD	teens	face & shoulder weakness
Limb-girdle	AR	teens–20s	hip weakness
Myotonic	AD	teens–20s	cramps, long face, distal weak
Emery-Dreifuss	XLR	child	contractures, cardiac block

Atrophy, contractures, weakness, scoliosis, respiratory failure, osteoporosis
Dx: EMG, muscle bx, serum CPK, dystrophin level

Congenital Myopathies

Central core myopathy	AD	hip dysplasia
Nemaline myopathy	AD	resp weakness, cardiomyopathy
Myotubular myopathy	AR/XLR	seizures, ptosis/resp weakness
Congenital fiber disproportion	varied	hip dysplasia, ↓ height & weight

Metabolic myopathy
(generally AR, ↑ CPK)

V	McArdle's	Phosphorylase deficiency
VII		Phosphofructokinase deficiency
II	Pompe's	Acid maltase deficiency
III		Debranching enzyme deficiency

Endocrine Myopathy: ↑↓T4, ↑↓PTH
Inflammatory: Polymyositis, Dermatomyositis, Sarcoid
Infectious: Trichinosis, cysticercosis, HIV
Toxic: Etoh, Meds (vincristine, chloroquine, steroids)

Steroid Myopathy:
Weakness starts with hips & prox LE, then prox UE, then distally when severe.
Starts weeks to years after steroid exposure. Normal CK.
EMG: No spontaneous activity, small polyphasic potentials, early recruitment.

Stroke

Risk factors: HTN, smoking, chol, ?obesity, LVH, CHF, Afib, DM
Non-modifiable - age, sex, race, previous CVA
Prevention: asa, plavix, coumadin
Thrombotic/Embolic, hemorrhagic, lacunar

Deficits:

- Loss of motor control & strength with synergistic movements
- Loss of motor coordination & balance, Incontinence
- Spasticity, Loss of sensation, Dysphagia
- Language & communication (aphasia, aprosody)
- Apraxia – disorder of skilled movement
- Hemispatial neglect (visual & spatial inattention)

MCA: Upper division	**Lower division (uncommon)**
Contralateral: HP(U>L), HA, hemianopsia	Contralateral hemianopsia
Dysphagia, uninhibited bladder,	
Dominant: Broca's aphasia, Apraxia	Dom: Wernicke's aphasia
Non-Dom: Aprosody, visiospatial, neglect	Non-Dom: affective agnosia

ACA
Contralateral: HP(L>U), HA
Grasp reflex (groping), disconnection apraxia, akinetic mutism (abulia)

PCA
Hemisensory defect
Visual impairment/agnosia, memory deficit
Prosopagnosia (cannot recognize familiar faces)
Dyschromatopsia (altered color discrimination)
Alexia (inability to read) without agraphia

Brainstem stroke syndromes

Wallenberg's (Lateral medulla) Vertebral occlusion, cuts off PICA
Ipsi: hemi-ataxia, facial pain/temp, Horners
Contra: body pain/temp
Dysphonia, Dysphagia, Nystagmus

Locked In (bilateral basal pons) b/l HP,
CN palsy (sparing of upward gaze)

Millard-Gubler (Lateral pons)
Ipsi: 6th CN palsy, facial weakness
Contra: HP

Benedikt's (midbrain tegmentum)
Ipsi: 3rd CN palsy
Contra: pain/temp/
joint position/ataxia/chorea

Weber's (Medial basal midbrain)
Ipsi: 3rd CN palsy
Contra: HP

Claude Syndrome
Cerebellar ataxia
Ipsi: 3rd CN palsy

Lacunar Syndromes

Pure Motor	Internal Capsule, Basis pontis, Pyramids
Pure Sensory	Thalamus, Thalamocortical projections
Sensory-Motor	Internal Capsule & Thalamus
Dysarthria-Clumsy hand	Ant Internal Capsule, Pons
Ataxia/Hemiparesis	Corona Rad., Internal capsule, pons, cerebellum
Hemiballismus	Caudate head, Thalamus, Subthalamic nucleus

Traumatic Brain Injury

Closed head injury = dura intact. Open head injury = dura injured.
Penetrating head injury: ie gunshot, stab, missile
Acceleration & deceleration injury: ie MVA brain laceration below skull fx
Contusions: inferior frontal & anteior temporal lobes
Diffuse axonal injury: widespread stretching of axons 2° brain rotation
Intracranial hemorrhage (subdural, epidural, intracerebral)
Anoxic injury: ischemia 2° hypoxemia or ↓ perfusion, ie cardiac arrest.

Assessment: Glascow Coma Scale (see section)
Severe TBI: GCS 3–8. Coma 6-8 hours (no eye opening or cognition)
Moderate TBI: GCS 9–12. Combative or lethargic. (Inappropriate response)
Mild TBI GCS 13–15. Confused/disoriented. AKA "Concussion"
Persistent Vegetative State: Sleep-wake cycles & spontaneous respiration

EEG, Evoked potentials, Neuropsychological testing: predict outcome.

Recovery:

Coma→Eye opening→Sleep-wake cycles→command following→speech
Best predictor of regaining consciousness: duration, etiology, age of patient.

Post Traumatic Amnesia (PTA): Impaired ability to learn new info & retain memory with confabulation. No memory of coma & PTA.
Retrograde amnesia: memory gap of events prior to injury.
PTA-Agitation: confusion, labile emotion, motor hyperactivity, aggression.
↓ attention, inappropriate behavior.

Treatment for agitation: (r/o medical causes)
Environmental (↓ level of stimulation & cognitive complexity)
Try to avoid neuroleptics, benzo's which cause sedation & memory loss
Clomazepine, α-depressants (mildly sedating), Trazodone (serotonergic)
β-blockers

Complications: hydrocephalus, seizures, CN damage, SIADH, and all other complications as seen in stroke & immobility.

Spina Bifida

Spina Bifida Occulta: Bony defect. Failure of mesodermal closure.
Spina Bifida aperta: Bony defect plus extrusion of tissue . . . Subdivied:
Myelomeningocele: bone, meninges and spinal cord
Meningocele: bone and meninges
Lipomeningocele, Lipomeningomyelocele: Lipomas within defect.
Diastematomyelia: splitting of lower spinal cord with bone & cartilage.

Incidence: 0.6 per 1000 births. 2000 new cases each year.
Multifactorial cause: Environmental and genetics.
Prevention: Folic Acid 0.8mg/day & avoid heat
Dx: Ultrasound 14-16 wks, AFP 16-18 wks. C-section recommended.
Goals of back surgery: ↓ risk of infection, preserve neuro function, ↓ deformity of kyphoscoliosis if present

Motor level does not correlate well with x-rays, anatomical site or sensory
Bladder & Bowel dysfunction: VU reflux common. CIC ± meds. UDS.

Hydrocephalus: 90%. Enlarged ventricles.
Sxs: ↑ head size, vomiting, headache, somnolence, irritability
Tx: VP shunt
Infections: 12% risk per child. Staph Epi most common.
Obstruction: 50% in 1st year require revision.

Arnold Chiari II malformation: Nearly 100%. Caudal displacement of cerebellum with elongation and kinking of the 4th ventricle
Sxs: stridor, aspiration, central apnea (central ventilatory dysfunction-CVD) Upper airway obstruction, vocal cord paralysis.
Tx: Decompression laminectomy, revision of VP shunts.

Hydromyelia: 50–80%. Dilation of central canal.
Sxs: rapidly progressive scoliosis, UE weakness, spasticity
Tx: laminectomy, direct shunting.

Tethered Cord Syndrome: 11–15% after repair.
Sxs: progressive neuro deficit from traction on conus and cauda equina

Cerebral Palsy

Diverse disorders with non-progressive injury to the brain up to ~2 years.
Incidence: 2/1000 births
Risk factors: gest.age <32wks, weight <2500 gms, malformations, IVH
  Maternal: MR, Sz, ↑ T4.
  Perinatal: Anoxia, ischemia
  Postnatal: Anoxia, ischemia, infection (TORCH), trauma

Interventricular hemorrhage

Grade I	Isolated to germinal matrix, lateral ventricle.
Grade II	IVH with normal ventricular size.
Grade III	IVH with ventricular dilitation.
Grade IV	IVH with parenchymal hemorrhage.

Periventricular leukomalacia: white matter necrosis after resolution of IVH
Strong predictor of CP.

Sxs: ↑ muscle tone, spasticity, ↑ DTR's, motor delay

Spastic	Diplegic
Hypotonic	Quadraplegic
Dyskinetic (Athetoid, Choreiform, Ballistic, Ataxic)	Tetraplegic
	Hemiplegic

Persistent motor delays: rolling, combat crawling, W-sitting, bunny hopping
Patterned movements: scissoring, guarding-UE's, extensor posturing
Persistent primitive reflexes: ATNR, STNR, TLR, moro

Associated complications:
  Ophtho: esotropia or exotropia require strabismus surgery.
  Oromotor: incomplete lip closure, poor suck, swallow
  Resp: aspiration, ineffective cough, restrictive lung disease
  GI: GE reflux, emesis, malnutrition, constipation
  Bladder & bowel: hyperreflexia & DESD most common.
  Mental retardation: ~30%. Severity correlates with motor deficit.
  Seizures: ~30%. Severity correlates with motor deficit.

Musculoskeletal:

Unbalanced spasticity and weakness contribute to deformity.
Coxa valgus, malformed femoral head, shallow acetabula→hip subluxation
Spine: scoliosis, kyphosis, rotational deformity.
Feet: calcaneovalgus (varus), pes cavus, hyperpronation, rocker-bottom

Treatment:

Common orthopaedic procedures:

Hip flexor lengthening (iliopsoas, rectus femoris, sartorius)
Hip adductor lengthening (adductor longus, gracilis)
Hamstring lengthening (medial, lateral)
Achilles tendon lengthening

Neurosurgical: dorsal rhizotomy
Botox injections: gastroc, hamstring (esp. medial), adductors
Chemolysis, intrathecal baclofen, Serial casting (see spasticity section)

Therapy: PT, OT, ST, feeding therapy
Therapy approaches: Bobaths, Rood, Ayres, Vojta, Domain-Delacato

Equipment: prone or supine standers, walkers, bathing equipment, wheelchairs, orthotics (tone reducing AFO's)

Prognosis:

Ambulation: 85% diplegic, 70% quadraplegic, most with hemiplegic.
Sit independently by 2 years correlates with eventual walking.
Not sitting by 4 years is a poor predictor of walking.

Primitive Reflexes

(Should normally be suppressed by time indicated)

ATNR (Asymmetric Tonic Neck Reflex): Turn head → Side faced extends and side turned away from flexes. (suppressed by 6 mo)

STNR (Symmetric Tonic Neck Reflex): If neck is extended → upper extremities extend and lower extremities flex. (>6 mo)

TLR (Tonic labyrinthine reflex): head position in space, supine position → extensor tone, prone position → flexor tone (4–6 mo)

Moro: sudden neck extension → arm ext/abd followed by flex/add (4–6mo)

Positive supporting: contact of sole → leg extension (3–7 mo)

Rooting: stoke corner of mouth → head/mouth/tongue turns toward (4 mo)

Palmar grasp: touch palm → flexing of fingers (5–6 mo)

Plantar grasp: touch soles (distal to MT heads) → toe flexion (12–18 mo)

Automatic neonatal walking: contact sole in vertical position and tilt body side to side → automatic alternating steps (3–4 mo)

Placing: tactile contact on dorsum of foot or hand → flexion to place the leg or arm over the object (1 year)

Snout reflex: tap lips → snouting

Crossed adductors: Lift vertically → legs adduct (10–12 mo)

Physiologic Postural Responses

(Should normally appear at time indicated and persist)

Head righting: visual & vestibular input → hold head upright (2–3 mo)

Body/Head righting: tactile & vestibular input → align body (4–6 mo)

Protective/propping: falling → extension of arm to prevent fall (5–12 mo)

Tilting: falling → adjustment of tone and posture to prevent fall (6-14 mo)

Segmental rotation: turn head → body follows in corkscrew (4-6 mo)

Landau: suspend in prone → neck, trunk & arms extend, legs flex (6 mo)

Parachute: sudden drop → legs and arms abduct (7-8 mo)

Rehabilitation of Rheumatic Disorders

Rheumatoid Arthritis

Common complications:
anemia, steroid myopathy, uncontrolled inflammation, quadraparesis (atlanto-axial subluxation),amputation, vasculitis, peripheral neuropathy, foot drop (mononeuritis multiplex), tendon rupture, joint effusions/synovitis

Common deformities:
- Boutonniere (DIP-ext, PIP-flex)
- Swan-neck (DIP-flex, PIP-ext)
- Ulnar deviation & subluxation
- Ruptured tendons
- MCP subluxation
- Subcutaneous nodules

X-rays: Soft tissue swelling, demineralization, uniform joint space narrowing, marginal erosions, deformities.

Goals of rehab: pain relief, ↑ ROM, ↑ strength, ↑ endurance, prevent and correct deformities, energy conservation, education and assistive devices.
Caution: over-exercising joints can cause flare-ups.

Pain relief: moist heat, NSAIDS, splints, immobilization, paraffin.
Splints: knees, wrists, AFO's, plastazote shoes

Osteoarthritis

Bouchard's nodes (PIP)
Heberden's nodes (DIP)
Hallux valgus, hallux rigidis, hammer toes
Osteophytes and symmetrical degeneration of:
- Shoulders: acromioclavicular >> glenohumeral
- Elbows, hips, knees, 1st CMC & MCP (thumb spica splint)
- Cervical & lumbosacral spine → stenosis, radic., myelopathy

X-rays: subchondral sclerosis, asymmetrical narrowing of the joint spaces, osteophyte formation, and bone cysts. Joint contour is wavy. Lateral subluxation of DIP or 1st CMC in advanced cases.

Ankylosing Spondylitis

Enthesopathy and synovitis primarily in the spine and sacroiliac joints.
Spine develops syndesmophytes and eventually a bamboo spine.
Iritis, aortic valve disease. HLA-B27 association.
Exercise, bracing and medications do not change the coarse of disease.
Keep the spine functional and allow it to stiffen in extension.
Exercise: push-ups, walking into corners with arms out.
Other joints may be involved. Mild trauma may cause spine fx.
Post operative heterotopic ossification after hip replacement is very common and may require prophylactic radiation therapy.

Psoriatic Arthritis

Tendonitis, enthesitis, synovitis may present in 5 major forms:
- Asymmetrical oligoarthritis
- Symmetrical arthritis with erosions
- Arthritis of the DIP joints primarily
- Spondylitis
- Arthritis mutilans

Tx: high toe box shoes, intra-articular steroids, splinting, paraffin baths

Scleroderma

Abnormal collagen with thickening of the skin
GI dysmotility, restrictive lung disease, pericardial restriction, myopathy.
Vasculitis, Raynaud's, dysphagia
CREST: calcinosis, Raynaud's, Esophageal dysfunction, sclerodactyly, telangiectasia

Tx: prevent contractures, strengthening, swallowing evaluation and modification of technique and consistency.

Dermatomyositis/Polymyositis

Proximal muscle strengthening and treatment of joint disease

Lupus

Non-erosive deforming arthritis. Functional splinting

Orthopaedic Rehabilitation

Weight bearing status is usually decided on by the surgeon or agreed upon by both surgeon and physiatrist.
In general, cemented, well fixated and well calcified bone, is allowed unrestricted weight bearing.
When there is a complicated fracture, displacement, unstable bone, severe osteopenia or cementless hardware, a more restricted weight bearing status is used and progress is based on callous formation on x-ray or after an appropriate amount of time has elapsed.
Bone typically takes 6 weeks to heal in a healthy individual and may be used to guide advancement of weight bearing status.

FWB = full weight bearing, unrestricted
WBAT = weight bearing as tolerated
PWB = partial weight bearing, 30%, 50%, etc.
TTWB = toe touch weight bearing, only rest toe on ground.
NWB = non weight bearing

If a restricted weight bearing status cannot be maintained by the patient due to cognitive deficiency, poor balance, etc., then the patient should be made non-weight bearing with bedside therapy only.

Methods of prosthestic fixation:

Polymethylmethacrylate (bone cement)
Porous coated – bony ingrowth
Hydroxyapatite coating
Press-fit stabilization

Total Hip Replacement

THR: both femoral head and acetabulum are replaced
Hemiarthoplasty: only femoral head replaced.
Lateral approach: gluteus medius and greater trochanter are divided
Posterior approach: extensors and short external rotators are divided.
Ambulation started in 1–2 days if WBAT
↑ risk of DVT, use prophylaxis, monitor for peroneal nerve palsy.
No resistive exercise for 6–8 wks.

Precautions: No flexion beyond 90°, internal rotation, adduction.
Adductor pillow/wedge when in bed or chair. Knee extension splints in bed,
sensory precautions
Cemented = WBAT, Cementless = TTWB x 6–8wks.
Avoid trauma & joint stress. Coumadin, cardiac (if needed)

PT: A/AAROM.
Isometric: Straight leg raises, quad & glut sets, abduction
Isotonic: ankle pumps, 4 point exercise, supine abd/add.
Stretching: gluts, quads, hams, gastrocs., Thomas stretch (hip flexors)
Stationary bike with high seat (min tension, 15mph, 2-4x/d)
Teach hip precautions. Bed mobility, transfer training, progressive ambulation training with AD (RW then SC). Improve standing balance in static/dynamic ranges. Wheelchair mobility and parts management. Community ambulation, stairs, ramps, curbs. Body mechanics, fall recovery, safety eval, car transfers, HEP, modalities for pain control.

OT: ADL/adaptive equipment, long handle equipment. Elevated toilet seat, tub chair, high chair, elevated mattress. Hip precautions. Joint protection, energy conservation. Standing balance for functional mobility. A/AAROM, isotonic PRE's, HEP, safety eval, kitchen training.

RT: arts/crafts, cooking, sewing, activity to improve standing tolerance/balance/endurance. Maintain hip precautions during activities. Social integration.

Total Knee Replacement

Full weight bearing within 1–2 days usually.
Constant passive motion (CPM) within 48 hours.
Gradually increase degree of flexion as tolerated.
If <90° flexion within 3 weeks, consider manipulation under anesthesia.
Non-cemented prostheses cannot fully weight bear for 6–8 wks.
No resistive exercise for 6–8 wks.

Precautions: falls, balance, avoid joint stress, coumadin,
Cemented = WBAT, Cementless = TTWB x 6–8wks.

PT: A/AAROM to LE's.
Isometrics: straight leg raises, quad sets.
Isotonic: ankle pumps, hip abd/add
Stretching program for quads, hams, gastrocs, hips.
CPM (no more than 40° for 1st 3 days, than ↑ 5–10°/day)
Body mechanics, improve standing tolerance & balance in static/dynamic ranges, bed mobility, transfer training, progressive amb training with RW,
Ambulate with knee immobilizer until able to do 3 straight leg raises
Patellar mobilization (POD 3–5)
Community ambulation, stairs, ramps, curbs. Fall recovery techniques. Wheelchair mobility and parts management. HEP, safety training.

OT: ADL, adaptive equipment, (long handle equipment)
Joint protective & energy conservation techniques.
A/AAROM to UE's Isotonic/isometric PRE's with static stretching.
HEP, safety training. Kitchen eval.

TR: Improve socialization, increase standing tolerance/balance/endurance during activities. Cooking group.

Other Arthroplasty

Shoulder Arthroplasty

Usually perform total joint arthroplasty with intact rotator cuff and hemiarthroplasty for arthritic patients with severe rotator cuff tears, complex fractures of the proximal humerus.

Performed to relieve pain. Usually does not ↑ ROM significantly.

Immediate post op ROM

Precautions: no extension past neutral, no external rotation past 90°

No active abduction or flexion until 4–6 weeks post op.

Avoid marked flexion and abduction.

Progressive resistive internal/external rotation with elbow at side.

Complications: humeral fx, axillary or suprascapular nerve injury, instability/dislocation, rotator cuff tear, RSD, infection

Goals: reach hand to mouth, face, scalp for hygiene, pain free shoulder

Elbow Arthroplasty

Constrained: original hinge type prosthesis

Semiconstrained: allow 8–10° of varus-valgus and axial toggle

Performed to reduce pain and allow hand to mouth.

Full ROM is usually not possible post op.

Gentle movement. No resistive exercise for 6–8 wks.

CPM if available.

No lifting >1 lb for 3 months. No lifting >5 lbs forever.

1st CMC Arthroplasty:

Used in rheumatoid arthritis with disabling destruction of the base of the thumb. Bone is removed to allow 1st MC to assume an abducted position.

May use a hemiarthroplasty (Swanson) with a single stem inserted into the 1st metacarpal using either concave or convex surface.

Brace in adduction for 5–6 weeks before starting movement.

Hip Fracture Rehabilitation

Garden Classification of subcapital (femoral neck) fractures
Stage I: Incomplete.
Stage II: complete oblique fx, non-displaced.
Stage III: complete with partial displacement, posterior cortex is compressed but not collapsed.
Stage IV: complete with full displacement, completely detached, limb in full external rotation.

Stage I & II can usually be reduced with 3 pins through the femoral neck.
Stage III & IV usually require a hemiarthroplasty due to ↑ risk of AVN

Intertrochanteric fx: (Generally heals well. ORIF with nail ± plate)
Type I: stable, non-displaced, trochanters not involved
Type II: (most common) displaced, varus deformity, medial cortex intact.
Type III: Vertically displaced with comminution of medial cortex, unstable
Type IV: intertrochanteric fx with subtrochanteric component

Day 1: Begin quad, hams, gluts sets & ankle pumps. Gentle active assisted abduction/ adduction. Supine leg slides. Bed mobility. Theraband for UE & PNF with therapist.

Day 2: Add more strengthening exercise, bed mobility, supine to sit transfers, start ambulation within weight bearing +RW

Day 3–7: start straight leg raises, lying & standing, if WBAT start weight shifting & minisquats, Daily Thomas stretch of anterior capsule and hip flexors, eval for assistive devices, sit-stand transfers, progressive ambulation BID.

Week 1–2: sets of quads, gluts, ankle pumps, hip & knee AROM (hip slides in supine), supine abduction, progressive straight leg raises. Add standing hip abduction, adduction, extension and flexion with hip & knee flexion exercises. 4 point exercise. Progress to cane once Trendelenburg lurch has resolved & gluteus medius is strong. Stationary bike, pool, treadmill.

IV

Diagnosis and Treatment of Pain

Shoulder Pain

3 synovial joints: glenohumeral, acromioclavicular, sternoclavicular
2 sliding surfaces: spaculothoracic, acromiohumeral

May be referred from cervical radic, trigger points, cardiac, viscera, pleura.

Degenerative arthritis: usually AC joint with tenderness & pain in adduction.
Regional pain sydrome: See RSD
Fx of clavicle: usually traumatic
Fx of proximal humerus: Surgical neck most common (axillary n. injury)

Dislocation: Anterior most common (>90%)
Hill-Sachs lesion (compression wedge fx of posterolateral humeral head)
Posterior: Bankart lesion
+Apprehension test: abd & ER causes anxiety

Subacromial bursitis	All clinically similar. Abd pain 60–120°
Supraspinatus tendonitis	Overuse or trauma. Pain worse at night.
Partial rotator cuff tear	Atrophy 2° disuse. Subacromial tender.
Painful arc syndrome	+ Hawkins: Abd,IR → pain
	+ Neer: Resisted forward flex → pain

Tx: rest, NSAIDS, modalities (ie U/S), shoulder exercise program
Injection: dorsal-lateral approach into subacromial bursa (lido+steroid)
Rotator cuff tear: +drop arm test: sudden drop after lowering arm ~90°

Bicipital tendinitis: Ant tenderness with pressure & IR/ER
+Yergeson's: pain with resisted supination
+Speeds: Forward flex shoulder against resistance

Biceps rupture: Bulge in biceps with weakness
Adhesive capsulitis: pain & limited ROM. Obliteration of axillary fold.
Calcific tendonitis: pain & limited ROM with calcific deposits

X-rays: AP, axillary, Groshe view (scapular plane), Y view (glenoid plane)
Consider arthoscopy, arthography, MRI

Elbow Pain

Supracondylar fx of the humerus: Most common in children
Dislocation: may accompany fx of olecranon or coronoid process.
Intra-articular fxs: immobilize for short time. ORIF for fx fragments.
Fx neck of radius: most undisplaced & impacted.
Epiphyseal injuries: early ORIF to prevent premature closure of plate.
Collateral ligaments: sprain & strain. X-ray to r/o fx with stress views.
Nursemaid's elbow: subluxed head of radius by forceful pull in children.
Biceps tendon rupture: at the elbow is rare.

Lateral epicondylitis: "tennis elbow", overuse. Inflammation of lateral collateral ligament, common extensor tendon, periosteum.
Resisted extension of wrist with supination causes pain.
Tx: rest, ergonomic modification to prevent recurrence, NSAIDS, U/S.
Injection of lido+steroid. Epicondylar splint if need to continue activity.

Medial epicodylitis: similar involving flexor tendons. (golfers, pitchers)

Osteochondritis dissecans: (Panner's disease) avascular necrosis of the capetellum. Pain, swelling & locking of elbow.

Olecranon Bursitis: (Student's elbow) repetitive trauma & inflammation

Rheumatoid arthritis: May involve the elbow joint. Pain, stiffness, swelling, rheumatoid nodules.
Degenerative arthritis: Uncommon, but may occur after trauma.
Septic arthritis: Less common than knee. Staph, Gonococci, pseudomonas.

Heterotopic ossification: Occurs in soft tissues around the elbow after manipulation, supracondylar or intercondylar fractures.

Hand and Wrist Pain

Always consider in the differential diagnosis: cervical radiculopathy, RSD, compartment syndrome, cardiac etiology, brachial plexus injury.

Sprains & strains
Infection/cellulitis

Carpal tunnel syndrome: median nerve compression, numbness/ tingling at night time, clumsiness, pain.
+Phalen's: flex wrist x 1min causes numbness
+Tinnel's: taping on wrist causes numbness.

DDx: cervical radiculopathy, peripheral neuropathy, TIA
Tx: NSAIDS, steroid injection, neutral wrist splint, surgical release

Fractures:

Distal end of radius: Colles' Fx (points dorsal), Smith's Fx (points palmar)
Scaphoid Fx: May lead to avascular necrosis. Snuff box tenderness.
Bennett's Fx: 1st MC near base and extends into joint. Requires ORIF.

DeQuervain's Tenosynovitis: Inflammation of tendon sheath of APL, EPB.
Pain and swelling over radial aspect of wrist near styloid.
+crepitus, +Finkelstein's: fingers flexed over thumb with forced adduction
Tx: rest, NSAIDS, steroid injection, thumb spica immobilizer

Osteoarthritis: most common in DIP's and CMC/MCP of thumb.
+morning stiffness for a few minutes on waking which decreases with activity.
1st CMC: pain in all movements, swelling more distal than DeQuervain's.

Hand and Wrist Pain *(cont.)*

Ganglion: benign cystic swelling most common over dorsal wrist

Dupuytren's contracture: palmar aponeurosis contracts causing flexion deformities of the digits. Related to DM, trauma, alcohol.

Trigger finger: painful finger locking and snapping with nodule. Tx: steroid injection and/or surgical release of sheath

Hip Pain

Hip flexion contracture: +Thomas's test: flex 1 hip all the way to eliminate lumbar lordosis and observe other leg elevation.

Congenital dislocation: Barlow & Ortolani's test for instability. If treated appropriately before child starts to walk, >95% develop normally.

Fractures:
Femoral Neck: pin (non-displaced) or hemiarthroplasty (displaced)
Intertrochanteric: Generally heals well. ORIF with nail ± plate

Dislocations: posterior most common. Consider sciatic nerve injury.
Tx: closed reduction under anesthesia or ORIF

Trochanteric bursitis: Bursa separates trochanter & gluteus maximus.
+Patrick-Fabere test: flex, abduct, ER, place foot on knee and push down.
Causes pain in bursitis, but also any SI joint pathology
Tx: NSAIDS, rest, steroid injection, stretch iliotibial band.

Iliopsoas bursitis: pain in groin and anterior thigh

Ischial bursitis: "weaver's bottom". Between ischial tuberosity & glut max.
Pain on sitting.

Snapping hip: may be caused by thickened posterior border of iliotibial band, trochanteric bursitis, irregular greater trochanter.

Osteoarthritis: Night pain & functional limitation are indications for THR.

Transient Synovitis: Effusion and synovitis. Self limited. Boys 3–10 years.

Slipped Capital Femoral Epiphysis: adolescent boys. Epiphysis is displaced inferiorly and posteriorly leading to coxa vara and sometimes AVN.
Tx: Traction, internal fixation, osteotomy.

Hip Pain *(cont.)*

Legg-Calve-Perthes disease (osteochondrosis): boys age 4–12. Blood supply to femoral head is compromised leading to deformed enlarged femoral head (coxa plana) with thick femoral neck. Early DJD.

Avascular necrosis of the femoral head: Assoc. with femoral neck fx, steroids, alcohol, sickle cell disease, caisson disease, gout, Gaucher's.

Knee Pain

Meniscal tear: McMurray's test: supine, knee 90°. Extend with valgus + ER stress→click
Apley grind: prone, knee 90°. Press down heel + rotation→pain
May cause loose body with pain & locking

Ligament tear: Pivot shift: supine, knee 70°, tibia IR & ext + valgus stress→lateral tibial condyle subluxes anteriorly with a clunk ~20-30° (tear of ACL or post. LM)
Drawer sign: supine, knee 90°. Sit on foot. Excessive ant movement (ACL)
Lachman's: same with knee at 20° and foot elevated
Varus & valgus stress: 0° & 20° for MCL, LCL tears

Bursitis: Prepatellar: overlying patella (housemaid's knee)
Infrapatellar: below patella. superficial and deep bursas. (clergyman's knee)
Anserine bursa: gracilis, semitendinosis, sartorius

Patellar fracture: comminuted or transverse most common.
May lead to early degeneration of the patellofemoral joint.

Patellar dislocation: predisposed by ↑ Q∠ (ASIS-patella-tibial tubercle)
Vastus medialis weakness, ligament laxity, patella alta (high riding)
Apprehension sign: laterally displace patella with flexion→anxiety

Chondromalacia patellae: "softening of the cartilage",anterior pain ± locking

Jumper's knee: partial patellar tendon tear at lower pole

Quadraceps rupture: Sudden severe pain and weakness.

Osteochondritis Dissecans: avascular necrosis of subchondral bone.
May cause a loose body in joint.
Adolescents & young adults.

Osgood-Schlatter's disease (tibial tubercle apophysitis):
10–15 years
Self limiting. Pain over tubercle with running, jumping, kneeling.

Consider: Septic arthritis, rheumatoid arthritis, osteoarthritis

Foot and Ankle Pain

Ligament Injury:

Inversion→Ant Talo-Fib > CalcFib > Post Talo-Fib.
Grade I: stretching without tear, stable
Grade II: incomplete tear + laxity
Grade III: complete tear
Dx: +anterior drawer, +inversion stress test, x-ray to r/o fx.
Tx: PRICE, cold ACE wraps, Unna boot or air splint, Taping, pain control
After inflammation improves: ROM, proprioceptive training, ↑ weight bearing, strengthening, if unstable→cast x 4 weeks or surgical repair

Achilles tendon rupture: sudden severe pain and weakness. +Thompson's test: prone, knee 90°. Squeeze calf→foot does not flex.

Rheumatoid arthritis: Most commonly affects MTP & PIP joints, tendon sheaths of TA, TP, FHL, peronei, retrocalcaneal bursa.

Plantar Fasciitis: medial and anterior heel pain. May see bone spur. Tx: good shoes/orthotics, stretching, NSAIDS, steroid injection, surgery, ice

Morton's neuroma: Burning pain of metatarsals radiating to the toes (metatarsalgia) 2° neuroma of digital nerves. Tx: good shoes, rest, steroid injection, surgical excision.

March fracture: metatarsal stress fx. Tx: rest, walking cast.

Deformities: caused by tight shoes, cavus foot, neurological conditions such as weakness of instrinsics, and peripheral neuropathy.
Mallet toe: DIP flexion
Hammertoe: PIP flexion
Clawing: hyperextension of MTP with flexion of PIP,DIP
Hallux Valgus: 1st MT head laterally displaced, bursa & callous.
Tx: stretching, splinting, good shoes, excision arthroplasy or osteotomy.
Hallux rigidus: ↓ movement in 1st MTP 2° ↓ joint space & osteophytes

Foot and Ankle Pain *(cont.)*

Club foot (Congenital Talipes equinovarus): plantarflex, inv. & add. of the forefoot.
Subluxation of talonavicular joint.
Tx: splinting, triple arthrodesis

Lumbosacral Spine Pain

Herniated Disc: L4-L5 most common
↑ pain & radiation with sitting, forward bending, coughing, sneezing, lifting
Straight leg test: +back & radiating leg pain 40–70°
Tx: rest, heat, analgesics, traction

Facet joint degeneration: joint space narrowing with osteophytes. May press on nerve.
Back pain may radiate down to foot, usually worse in morning, stiffness. Pain with extension of spine.
Tx: rest, heat, NSAIDS, corset, exercise, steroid injection.

Spinal Stenosis: pain & weakness of legs with walking esp. up-hill. "neurogenic claudication", extension causes worsening of stenosis,
Tx: NSAIDS, strengthen abdominals, corset in flexion, trial of steroid injection for soft tissue swelling, surgical decompression.

Spondylolysis: defect in pars interarticularis, usually asymptomatic
Spondylolisthesis: forward slipping. Dull aching low back pain.
Tx: NSAIDS, isometric exercise, corset, surgery (grade III & IV)

Myofascial Pain Syndrome: Trigger point injection.
Muscle & ligament strain and overuse.
Consider Spondyloarthropathies, osteomyelitis, bony mets (night pain), aortic aneurysm, pelvic pathology, hip DJD, osteoporosis, vertebral fracture (usually thoracic)
Investigations: x-rays, EMG/NCS, CT, MRI, bone scan, myelogram.
Often diagnosis is difficult to make. A trial of conservative management is usually appropriate to start with.
Short bed rest, NSAIDS to

Lumbosacral Spine Pain *(cont.)*

control pain & inflammation, narcotics if severe.
Muscle relaxants, massage, local heat, traction, trigger point injections,
If failed conservative management, then consider . . . corsets & braces,
Medrol dose pack, epidural injections, intradiscal chymopapain,
intradiscal electrothermy-IDET, laser decompression-PLDD

Cervical Spine Pain

Whiplash: flexion-extension acceleration with soft tissue injury. Muscles & ligaments are stretched and may cause tearing. Neck & head pain with muscle spasm, limited ROM
Tx: soft collar, ice (first few days), heat, NSAIDS, muscle relaxants, ROM

Atlanto-axial subluxation in Rheumatoid arthritis: May give rise to occipital neuralgia, vertebral artery compression (loss of balance)

Degenerative arthritis: There is often a mixture of disc degeneration with loss of height, osteophytes of facet joints & uncovertebral joints, narrowing of the intervertebral foramina.

Radiculopathy: may be caused by disc herniation or foraminal stenosis from osteophytes. Pain may radiate down arm esp. with extension, lateral flexion and lateral rotation. C6 & C7 most commonly involved.

Cervical myelopathy: With more involvement, may develop difficulty walking, heavy legs, bladder dysfunction, ↑ LE tone & DTR's, ↓ sensation.

Tx: heat, traction, ROM, NSAIDS, muscle relaxants (for spasms), trigger point injections, cervical collar, decompression (rarely needed).

Cervical Spine Pain *(cont.)*

Thoracic Outlet syndrome: compression of neurovascular bundle over cervical rib or C7 ligamentous structure as it passes between anterior and middle scalenus. May be caused by drooped shoulders, congenital narrowing, Pancoast's tumor, hyperabduction of the arm.

Gradual onset, young-middle aged women. May cause numbness & tingling of the 4th and 5th digits and medial forearm, worse at night. Intrinsic muscle weakness in advanced cases.+Adson's maneuver: hyper-extend neck, rotate to side of symptoms & hold a deep breath, abduct arm and compare radial pulses. Weakened pulse or reproduction of numbness/tingling is positive.

Also consider: Ankylosing spondylitis, infections, trigger points, peripheral neuropathy, primary tumors, mets.

Pain Pharmacotherapy

Acetaminophen: analgesic & antipyretic. Few side effects. Max 4gm/d
Overdose usually >10gms/day can lead to hepatic failure.

Ultram: opiate like analgesic 50–100mg q4–6 hrs. Avoid in opiate dependant

NSAIDS: anti-inflammatory, analgesic, antipyeritc.
SE: renal, GI ulceration, gastritis, bleeding. HTN, CHF exacerbation.
↑ levels of methotrexate, lithium, phenytoin, digoxin, cyclosporin.

Salicylates: Asprin, Salflex, Dolobid
Proprionic acids: Ansaid, Ibuprofen, Orudis, Naprosyn, Daypro
Acetic acids: Voltaren, Lodine, Indocin, Toradol, Relafen, Clinoril, Tolectin
Others: Feldene, Meclomen
COX2: Celebrex: OA: 100mg qd-bid, RA: 200mg qd-bid
Vioxx: OA: 12.5–25mg qd, Acute pain: 50mg qd

Narcotic/NSAID combinations:
With acetaminophen: Anexsia, Tyl#3 & 4, Darvocet, Fioricet, Lorcet, Lortab, Percocet, Roxicet, Talacen, Tylox, Vicodin, Wygesic, Zydone
With ASA: Darvon, Empirin, Fiorinal, Percodan, Soma

Narcotic	Equiv. IV	IV:PO	Start Dose	Half-life
Short half-life Opioids				
Morphine	10mg	1:3	15–30mg q3–4	$2^1/_2$–3 hr
Hydromorphone (Dilaudid)	1.5mg	1:5	4–6mg q3-4	2–3 hr
Codeine	130mg	$1:1^1/_2$	30–60mg q3–4	$2^1/_2$–3 hr
Oxycodone	*(1:1 with PO Morphine)*		5–10mg q3–4	2–3 hr
Meperidine (Demerol)	75mg	1:4	50mg q3–4*	3 hr
Oxymorphone	1mg	–	5mg PR	$1^1/_2$ hr
Fentanyl patch*	100ug	–	25 µg/hr	
Long half-life Opioids				
Methadone	10mg	1:2	5–10mg q4–8	12–150 hr
Levorphanol	2mg	1:2	2–4mg q4–8	15 hr

**Not recommended for starting*

Electrodiagnostics

Nerve conduction basics: Stimulate a nerve and record response at a distant site, either along the same nerve (sensory) or muscle (motor). A supramaximal stimulus is needed to produce a maximal wave. Active electrode (G1) and reference electrode (G2) are placed ~4 cm apart.

Sensory Nerve Conduction Study

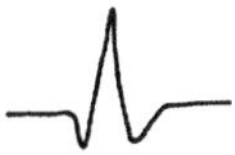

Sensory nerve action potential (SNAP).
Stimulate & record pure sensory nerve.
(i.e. Sural)
Stimulate mixed nerve & record distally over cutaneous branch (antidromic)
Stimulate cutaneous nerve & record proximal mixed nerve (orthodromic)
Antidromic SNAP's are larger & easier to get than orthodromic.
Usually triphasic potentials with initial small positive (down) reflection.
Amplitude: measure of the number of axons that conducted and usually measured from peak to peak in microvolts *(uV)*.
Latency: time it takes *(msec)* to travel along nerve, usually measured from stimulus to the negative peak.
Conduction velocity: Distance divided by the difference between proximal & distal latency *(m/sec)*.

Motor Nerve Conduction Studies

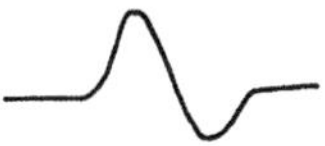

Compound Muscle Action Potential (CMAP)
Stimulate nerve and record over muscle belly.
Represents the summation of all motor axons, neuromusclar junction and muscle fibers.
Biphasic wave with large initial negative phase (up)
Amplitude: measure of number of axons, measured from baseline to negative peak in millivolts *(mV)*.
Area: Total area under curve. Longer traveled distance results in shorter wider curve (temporal dispersion), but area should be preserved.
Distal Latency: time *(msec)* from stimulus to initial negative take off.
Conduction velocity: Distance divided by the difference between proximal & distal latency *(m/sec)*.

Electrodiagnostics *(cont.)*

F-wave latency: Stimulate mixed nerve & record over muscle. (8–10 times) Potential travels proximally to anterior horn cell and then back down axon to muscle. Should see a variety of waveforms, since different axons are stimulated each time. (Useful for proximal nerve lesions)

Tibial H reflex: Stimulate mixed tibial nerve at popliteal fossa & record at soleus muscle. (8–10 times) Start at very low gain and slowly increase since H reflex is abolished once CMAP comes in.

Needle EMG

Insertional activity: Burst of muscle action potentials when inserting a needle. May be increased in denervated muscles, myotonic disorder and decreased in muscle replacement with fat or paralysis.

Spontaneous activity: Resting needle recording activity is abnormal, except in end plate.
Fibrillations: brief spikes (sounds like raindrops on a tin roof).
Positive sharp waves: small biphasic waves with downward deflection.
Fasciculations: Spontaneous large motor units. (seen in ALS)
Myotonia, myokymia, complex repetitive discharges.

Voluntary activity: Patient flexes muscle and you record motor unit potentials (MUP's)

Recruitment: Normally, ↑ effort results in initiation of more MUP's and a faster firing rate.

Reduced recruitment: rapid firing rate of a small number of MUP's. Caused by any disorder that affects axons or muscle fibers.

Poor activation: decreased number of MUP's and slow firing rate.

Early recruitment: Many motor units firing during minimal muscle contracture, seen in myopathies.

MUP duration: ↑ duration seen with sprouting in neuropathy with re-innervation of muscle. ↓ Duration seen in myopathy, NMJ disease.

MUP amplitude: ↑ amp seen in chronic neurogenic disorders (i.e. polio)

Electrodiagnostics *(cont.)*

MUP polyphasia: 5 or more phases. Seen in both myopathy & neuropathy after reinnervation.

Nerve compression: Affects both motor and sensory in the distribution of a peripheral nerve and can often be localized with several points of stim.

Conduction block (segmental demyelination): When myelin is lost after a compression injury and causes slowing, phase cancellation and temporal dispersion. This causes an apparent decrease in CMAP amplitude and/or area with proximal stimulation when compared to distal stimulation.

≥50% drop in CMAP amplitude with ≤15% prolonged duration, or
≥50% drop in CMAP area, or
≥30% drop in area and/or amplitude over a short segment.
Can occur in early axonal injury before Wallerian degeneration.

With pure demyelinating injury, prognosis is good with recovery in 2–3 months after remyelination occurs.

With Axonal injury: Wallerian degeneration causes loss of motor amplitude in 4–5 days and sensory amplitude in 8–11 days. Fibrillations start to occur in 2–3 weeks and neurogenic potentials start to be seen in 2–3 months. Prognosis is worse with improvement made through resprouting and reinnervation which may take years and may be incomplete.

Radiculopathy: Normal SNAPs in spite of subjective sensory loss. With axonal loss: low amplitude CMAP & fibs in segmental myotomal distribution of muscles and paraspinals, neurogenic MUP's, reduced recruitment. Large polyphasic MUP's may occur after 2–3 months. H reflex may be absent, low amplitude or slow velocity when compared to other side in S1 radiculopathy. F-wave asymmetry may exist. Site of lumbar herniation does not always correlate with involved root. May have a normal exam in pure demyelinating injury.

Plexopathy: Denervation of both motor and sensory in the distribution of the brachial or lumbosacral plexus. Paraspinals should be normal.

Peripheral Polyneuropathy: Symmetrical motor and sensory involvement with low amp, slow velocity in multiple nerves. May see fibrillations, neurogenic units, abnormal H-reflex & F-wave in advanced cases.

Upper Extremities Normal Values

Motor:

	Record	Amp	CV	DL	distance(cm)
Median	APB	≥4.0	≥49	≤4.4	7
Ulnar	ADM	≥6.0	≥49	≤3.3	7
Ulnar	FDI	≥7.0	≥49	≤4.5	8–12
Radial	EIP	≥2.0	≥49	≤2.9	4–6

Antidromic Sensory:

	Amp	CV	DL	distance(cm)
Median	≥20	≥50	≤3.5	13
Ulnar	≥17	≥50	≤3.1	11
Radial	≥15	≥50	≤2.9	10
Dorsal Ulnar cut	≥8	≥50	≤2.5	8
Lat antebrach cut	≥10	≥55	≤3.0	12
Med antebrach cut	≥5	≥50	≤3.2	12

Median-Palmar stim studies

	Sign palm/wrist amp ratio
Median motor: wrist→APB	>1.2
Median motor: palm→APB	
Median sensory: wrist→2nd digit	≥1.6
Median sensory: palm→2nd digit	

Erb's point stimulation:

	Record	DL	distance (cm)
Axillary	Deltoid	≤4.9	15–21
Musculocutaneous	Biceps	≤5.7	23–29
Suprascapular	Supraspinatus	≤3.7	7–12
Suprascapular	Infraspinatus	≤4.3	10–15

(From: Preston DC, Shapiro BE: Electromyography and Neuromuscular Disorders: Clinical-Electrophysiologic Correlations, 1998, Butterworth-Heinemann Medical, with permission)

Lower Extremities Normal Values

Motor:

	Record	Amp	CV	DL	distance(cm)
Peroneal	ADB	≥2.0	≥44	≤6.5	9
Peroneal	TA	≥5.0	≥44	≤6.7	5–10
Tibial	AH	≥4.0	≥41	≤5.8	9
Tibial	ADM	≥3.0	≥41	≤6.3	10

Antidromic sensory:

Sural	≥6	≥40	≤4.4	14
Superficial peroneal	≥6	≥40	≤4.4	14
Saphenous	≥4	≥40	≤4.4	14
Medial plantar	≥2	≥35		variable
Lateral plantar	≥1	≥35		variable

Mixed plantar nerve study:

Medial plantar	≥3	≥45	≤3.7	14
Lateral plantar	≥3	≥45	≤3.7	14

F wave: Upper extremity: 32
Lower extremity: 56

Craniobulbar studies:

Facial	Nasalis	≥1.0	≤4.2
Facial	Orbicularis	≥1.0	≤3.1

Blink reflex	Latency	side-to-side difference
R1 (ipsilateral)	≤13	≤1.2
R2 (ipsilateral)	≤41	≤5
R3 (contralateral)	≤44	≤7

(From: Preston DC, Shapiro BE: Electromyography and Neuromuscular Disorders: Clinical-Electrophysiologic Correlations, 1998, Butterworth-Heinemann Medical, with permission)

Index

R

S

T

U

W

Title List from International Medical Publishing

ISBN — Title — Author — Price

Intern Pocket Survival Guides

0-9634063-0-2 Intern Pocket Survival Guide–Masterson $7.50

0-9634063-1-0 CCU Intern Pocket Survival Guide–Masterson/Rothenhaus $7.50

0-9634063-2-9 ER Intern Pocket Survival Guide–Rothenhaus/Masterson $7.50

0-9634063-3-7 ICU Intern Pocket Survival Guide–Masterson/Rothenhaus/Tenner $7.50

0-9634063-5-3 Surgical Intern Pocket Survival Guide–Chamberlain $7.50

0-9634063-9-6 Oncology Intern Pocket Survival Guide–Tenner/Masterson/Rollhauser $7.50

1–883205–00–X The OB/GYN Intern Pocket Survival Guide $9.95

Emergency Handbooks

0-9634063-8-8 EKG Pocket Survival Guide–International Medical Publishing $6.00

1-883205-16-6 ACLS Pocket Survival Guide–International Medical Publishing $6.00

1-883205-19-0 PALS Pocket Survival Guide–International Medical Publishing $6.00

1-883205-46-8 Pocket Guide to Emergency and Disability Scores $6.00

1-883205-20-4 First Aid–Bureau of Mines $6.25

Clinical Practice Handbooks

1-883205-44-1 Pocketful of Prevention–Masterson $7.50

Medical Student Titles

0-9634063-6-1 Pocket Guide to Eponyms and Subtle Signs of Disease–Tenner/Masterson $7.50

0-9634063-4-5 Intern Pocket Admission Book–contains blank admit forms $4.00

1-883205-18-2 How to be a Truly Excellent Junior Medical Student–Lederman $12.00

U.S. Public Health Service and other federal agencies

1-883205-32-8 Clinician's Handbook of Preventive Services, 2nd ed.–USPHS $20.00

1-883205-13-1 Guide to Clinical Preventive Services, 2nd ed.–United States Preventive Services Task Force $24.00

1-883205-42-5 The JNC VI Report on Prevention, Detection, Evaluation, and Treatment of High Blood Pressure–NIH $8.95

1-883205-33-6 Health Information for International Travel 1996-97–CDC $14.95

1-883205-45-X 1998 Guidelines for Treatment of Sexually Transmitted Diseases–CDC $7.95

ORDER FORM

In addition to your address, please include an e-mail or phone number so that we might contact you with any questions about your order.

Name: ____________________

Address: ____________________

City, State, Zip: ____________________

Daytime phone/e-mail: ____________________

❑ Personal Check
❑ Credit Card (circle one): Visa Mastercard Amex Discover

Card Number ____________________

Expiration ____________________

Signature ____________________

Title	ISBN	Quantity	Price	Total
REHAB	1-58808-111-7		9.95	
		Tax 5.75% D.C.		
		S&H (see below)		
		Total		

Sales Tax 5.75% in Washington D.C.
Shipping charges are $5.00 for the first book, $.50 for each additional in the 48 continental states. Please call for other rates.
Please send your order to: Reiter's Scientific & Professional Books, 2021 K Street, N.W., Washington, D.C. 20006.
Information & ordering: 702-223-3327. Fax: 202-296-9103.
E-mail inquiries to: books@reiters.com
or visit us on the web at www.medicalpublishing.com.